Humanizing Health Care:
Alternative Futures for Medicine

Humanizing Health Care:
Alternative Futures for Medicine

Robert F. Rushmer

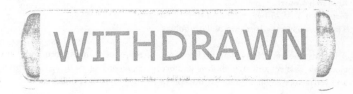

The MIT Press
Cambridge, Massachusetts, and London, England

Research for this book was supported in part by grants from the National Institute of General Medical Sciences (GM 16436-06) and the National Heart and Lung Institute (HL 07293-13). The manuscript was prepared in part during a Fellowship at the Seattle Battelle Research Center.
Copyright © 1975 by
The Massachusetts Institute of Technology

This book was set in CRT Baskerville
by The Colonial Press, Inc.,
printed on R and E Book
by Halliday Lithograph Corporation,
and bound in Columbia Millbank Linen MBL 4974
by The Colonial Press, Inc.,
in the United States of America.

Second printing, 1976

Library of Congress Cataloging in Publication Data

Rushmer, Robert Frazer, 1914–
  Humanizing health care.

  Includes bibliographical references and index.
  1. Medical care—United States. 2. Health planning—United States. I. Title.
[DNLM: 1. Delivery of health care—United States. 2. Health and welfare planning—United States. WA540 AA1 R95n]
RA395.A3R86   362.1′0973   75-1399
ISBN 0-262-18075-8

Contents

Preface

Health-care delivery in the United States has undergone revolutionary changes in the past quarter century, characterized by explosive expansions of information, specialization, sophisticated facilities, and costs. Like most other aspects of modern society health-care delivery systems are confronted by serious problems directly resulting from extraordinary technological successes and overabundance. It is no longer possible to seek the answers to current health problems by directing attention only to the health professions and their facilities. As societies have become more complicated and interactive, emerging problems have become so complex that their solutions demand mobilization and convergence of many different areas of knowledge and competence. For this reason it is increasingly important to take a long look with a wide perspective in assessing alternative solutions for our major problems. This book is designed to identify the major problems of health, to define the most pressing requirements and issues, and to consider viable mechanisms for achieving their solutions.

The nature and extent of the most serious problems of health-care delivery are well established and widely recognized. They have resulted from long traditions and evolutionary changes and include such factors as soaring costs, unavailability of care at particular times and places, complicated access to the system, large segments of the population lacking care, and maldistribution of health personnel and facilities. Confronting each of these problem areas are clearly visible obstacles to various remedies, so that the "next steps" are usually far from obvious. These uncertainties are compounded by the accelerating rates of change in almost all segments of society.

The current health-care system evolved with little or no long-range planning or direction. Our main hope for the future lies in our ability to understand our history, assess our current status, and undertake realistic long-range planning that will yield the highest probability for attaining livable or attractive futures. Since we lack historical precedents for these procedures, our learning and accomplishment must be simultaneous. This book is not designed to provide a blueprint, a pathway, or even a set of specific suggestions. Instead it is designed to demonstrate mechanisms by which problem areas can be more clearly recognized, the principal issues identified, and possible options evaluated in terms of advantages, disadvantages, and consequences. The proposed mechanisms take into account the close functional relationships between health-care delivery and other societal disciplines, such as economics, sociology, politics, education, communications, and ethics, and their specific priorities. In order that interested people in all these various walks of life may appreciate their own relationship to the problem a conscious effort has been made to avoid medical or technical jargon and to support the most fundamental concepts with schematic illustrations intended to convey their meaning at a glance. If these mechanisms provide a common point of discussion or departure for public-spirited people from the many disciplines involved in seeking attractive alternatives for bettering the national health, the effort will have been well rewarded.

Long-range planning for health has been almost completely neglected in preparations for the coming plunge into some form of nationwide insurance coverage. In Chapter 1 are presented some of the current trends in futures research and their limited application to the projection of future developments in health technology. A more promising approach is the "creation of desirable futures" attained by converting current objections into future objectives (Chapter 2). A wide variety of optional approaches to attain these goals can then be developed and assessed. If these desirable options are kept in mind, it should be possible to make subsequent decisions, policies, and legislation that can facilitate realization and rationalization of the most attractive alternatives. The assessment of alternative futures for health care demands consideration of the total health-care delivery mechanism as an interacting system. The nature and extent of responsibility for different types and severities of ailments must be defined by categories that can, in turn, be delegated to the public, to the medical sector, and to society as a whole. This process will clearly indicate the discrepancies between current capabilities and future needs.

Chapter 3 is devoted to cost/benefit relationships, which assume increasing importance whenever available resources become so strained that priorities must be established. Health professionals have not heretofore been required to defend or justify the costs of their services since health and life have always been held to be above any monetary value. This view is not tenable whenever some people are being deprived of health care for lack of available personnel, facilities, and services. Some possible methods of relating costs to the benefits of health care are proposed to illustrate the feasibility of applying this sort of analysis. The concept of the value added by patient contact with health professionals is also considered in terms of various levels of therapeutic effectiveness.

Present and prospective priorities are discussed in Chapter 4 to illustrate that a preponderance of available health resources are focused on a few "favored" categories of illness. Current preoccupation centers on the great killers, such as heart disease, stroke, cancer, and kidney failure, which are found predominantly among older age groups whose productive life expectancy can be extended only to a limited degree. The high technologies developed for these conditions are currently benefiting a relatively small proportion of the populace at enormous cost to the whole nation. Meanwhile the most prevalent causes of death, disability, and malfunction among the young and productive segments of society are being neglected to a tragic degree. Accidents, injuries, and violence, which are the prime threats to people younger than thirty years of age, are not being effectively managed because of nationwide deficiencies in our emergency systems. Priorities are discussed for different age groups, geographical locations, and racial groups, as well as for the mentally ill, senior citizens, and those facing impending death.

Chapters 5 and 6 present the major requirements for personnel, facilities, and organizational relationships for future health-care systems along with a large selection of attractive options for approaching or attaining these objectives.

The present and future importance of ambulatory and home-based care of the sick and handicapped is discussed at some length in Chapter 7. Potential mechanisms for developing not only substitutes for, but improved versions of, the traditional family physician are presented that would more fully utilize our highly developed communications and transportation systems.

Chapter 8 sets forth the concept that citizens must assume a greater degree of responsibility for their own health. More effective utilization of our communications systems should make it possible for many or most citizens to be much more fully informed concerning how to manage a larger selection of their ailments. A long-range objective could be to have a greatly increased segment of the population actively participating in both decisions about and management of individual illnesses with the aid and guidance of a wide variety of health professionals and paraprofessionals. The many attractive options are presented as a list of alternatives from which desirable futures can be forged, rather than as specific suggestions concerning what can and should be done.

Acknowledgments

The contributions of both Sue Walmsley and Joyce Gibson to the preparation of this manuscript are greatly appreciated. Several of the illustrations were prepared by Hedi Nurk. Allen Holloway contributed many valued suggestions and references. Thanks are due Drs. Herbert Sherman and Anthony Komaroff for providing both written material and illustrations for the section on health guides in Chapter 5. An opportunity to view some of the European health systems was accorded by a professional leave from the University of Washington during which I was a fellow of the Battelle Memorial Institute. I am grateful to Dr. Ron Paul, my sponsor, and my many helpful friends at Battelle/Frankfurt and Battelle/Geneva. My appreciation is also due to the Academic Press for their permission to reproduce portions of Chapter 7 which were published previously in *Advances of Biomedical Engineering*.

1
Projections of Future Developments in Health-Care Delivery

• A review of the history of medicine reveals that many different figures
have played central roles in the practice of medicine, beginning with
primitive native healers or "witch doctors" and passing through stages
involving clerics, barbers, philosopher-physicians, family doctors, and,
most recently, scientific specialists. Healers have held preferential and key
positions in most cultures. Many of our current medical traditions can be
traced to a mystique which allowed the healer to bring relief and
reassurance to patients even when he was incapable of directly affecting
the course of illness. The need for a close and understanding doctor-
patient relationship may be reduced when powerful and effective
treatments can cure or alleviate illness, but it remains very important for
the many and varied forms of illness still lacking effective therapy.

The traditional nineteenth-century image of the physician was that of a
kindly, sympathetic, unselfish, and dedicated man whose primary goal was
to bring comfort and care to his patients. Until the turn of this century the
standard treatment for many illnesses was to send the patient to bed and
submit him to some unpleasant procedure or prescription. In those days
the state of medical knowledge was such that home remedies prepared by
a grandmother or maiden aunt were often as effective as the complicated,
ineffectual concoctions of the pharmacist. The medicines of the day were
derived mainly from natural organic substances such as digitalis, quinine,
opium, and cascara. These organic materials and many others were
elaborately bottled, elegantly flavored, and carefully prescribed. Oliver
Wendell Holmes is reported to have stated that if 80% of these
prescriptions had been poured into the sea, only the fishes would have
suffered. Therapeutic measures were administered mainly to achieve
symptomatic relief.

• Increasing Effectiveness—Diminishing Satisfaction

At the turn of the century the country was supplied with a relatively large
number of doctors, many of whom had emerged with very limited training
from the "diploma mills" and had gained most of their competence

through apprenticeship and on-the-job training. Actually the number of doctors per 1,000 population was greater in 1900 than it is today, and they were at that time more widely distributed in rural areas than in urban America.[1] Hospitals were scarce, but they were not missed because most practice was conducted in the patient's home or the doctor's office. In those days there were always spinster aunts, young cousins, or neighbors to look after the aged, the feeble, the handicapped, the mentally deficient, and the chronically ill. So many people succumbed to acute illness that chronic illnesses were not nearly so prevalent as they are today.

The kindly old family doctor who served as counselor and source of concern and sympathy carved a lasting impression in people's minds. Nowadays the general public still expects the selfless dedication and ready availability of the old family doctor, but they would also like him to be armed with the best that modern medical science and technology can provide.

The accelerated progress in the prevention, cure, and management of many diseases and disabilities during this century, and particularly in the last two decades, is illustrated in Figure 1.1. The health of the nation has greatly benefited from improved nutrition through ready access to essential foods and vitamins. Public-health measures have been effective in eliminating or controlling many frightful epidemic and infectious diseases. The collection of large amounts of quantitative data for a variety of disease states has created a much more objective basis for diagnosis. In turn, the new diagnostic techniques have greatly added to the reliability, objectivity, and specificity of the patient's data base, particularly during the last 25 years.

Surgery has been aided by two major improvements, asepsis and anesthesia, in the last century. The original concentration of surgery on cutting-out or sewing-up has been refined and expanded to include increasingly sophisticated reconstructive surgery, artificial tissue substitutes, and, currently, the development of artificial substitutes for organ function. (An example is the heart-lung machine, which has allowed the meticulous repair of structures inside the heart.) A major contribution to survival following surgery has been made by the enormous improvement in postoperative management afforded by highly sophisticated intensive-care units.

PROGRESS IN HEALTH CARE

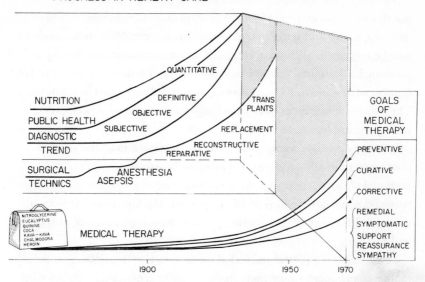

Figure 1.1 During the last century progress in health care has been phenomenal in all its phases, including nutrition, public health, diagnostic capability, and surgical techniques. Medical therapy has extended its goals from support and symptomatic relief to the correction, cure, and prevention of illness.

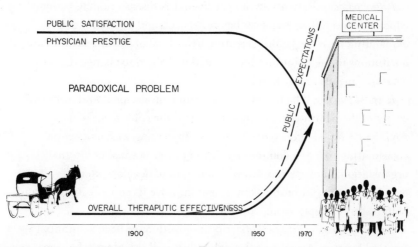

Figure 1.2 Paradoxically, the greatly increased ineffectiveness of medicine achieved by replacing the horse-and-buggy doctor with highly trained teams in medical centers has been accompanied by a precipitous drop in public satisfaction and physician prestige. This is attributable in part to public expectations overshooting the ability of health professionals to deliver.

This improved therapeutic effectiveness of medical care has made it possible to upgrade the goals of medical therapy. Conditions for which only supportive and symptomatic treatment was available in the past can now be remedied, alleviated, corrected, cured, and in some cases even prevented. Continued research and development is designed to expand the number of diseases and disabilities for which definitive care is available. The control of infections and the management of metabolic defects are notable examples.

Strangely enough, major improvements in the medical and surgical management of ailments have not produced corresponding public approval or satisfaction with the health-care delivery system. According to Anne Somers,[2] paradoxical problems pervade the four essential elements of the health-care delivery system, namely physicians, patients, hospitals, and finances:

Physician paradox. Better trained physicians in larger numbers are seeing more patients, performing more miracles, and earning more money than ever before, *but* an imbalance between supply and demand is producing emotional and financial pressures and a growing resentment and public depreciation of the medical profession.

Patient paradox. Patients are longer-lived, less disease-ridden, better educated, and richer than ever before, *but* rich and poor alike are demanding far more health care and are critical of existing health-care institutions to the point that they seem determined to change them by whatever means are at hand.

Hospital paradox. The hospital—the unique professional and technical center of the health-care world—still enjoys the confidence of most Americans, *but* it suffers partial paralysis in dealing with its essential coordinating role as a community health center because of internal organizational defects coupled with a failure to develop external organizational relationships that might improve its cost-effectiveness and help restrain steeply rising costs.

Financial paradox. Financial barriers to health have been substantially reduced for most Americans through public and private mechanisms (i.e., insurance and governmental subsidies) that benefit both providers and consumers, *but* the influx of money has added further financial pressures to soaring costs and, despite federal subsidies, those segments of the population that have the greatest need for health care are currently unable to pay for its benefits.

It seems ironic that during the present period, when medical, surgical, public-health, and nutritional aspects of health care have all witnessed their greatest achievements, the public's satisfaction has plummeted to new lows (Figure 1.2). There seems no doubt that the status and prestige of physicians was much higher when horse-and-buggy doctors were available day or night, dedicated public servants willing to make home calls. A doctor was then expected to be knowledgeable regarding the whole patient and his family, and to offer his services willingly and with little apparent regard for his own convenience, income, or well-being. In contrast the medical team functioning in a modern, sophisticated hospital or medical center is far more effective in actively alleviating disease and disability than "old doc" was. The public appreciation and enthusiasm for the enormously enhanced quality and expanded effectiveness of health care has been diluted by disenchantment with the manner in which it is administered. Many patients are convinced that some of their deeply felt needs, formerly satisfied by the country doctor or family physician, could be built into modern medical institutions by some reordering of priorities and restructuring of the system. At the same time exaggerated expectations have been engendered by much that modern patients see and hear through mass media.[3]

The technical accomplishments of "superspecialists" utilizing sophisticated equipment to prolong lives have been widely publicized but have actually benefited only a relatively small segment of the population. The less dramatic but much more common ailments to which mankind is subject will not likely be alleviated by dramatic innovations of the sort so prominently portrayed in newspapers or on television (Figure 1.3). New techniques have greatly increased our ability to predict the rate at which new technologies will be utilized for health care.

Some Techniques of Futures Research: Technological Forecasting

In the past few years futures research has become a small industry in the United States, involving approximately 3,000 full- and part-time workers. Many different disciplines are represented, including engineering,

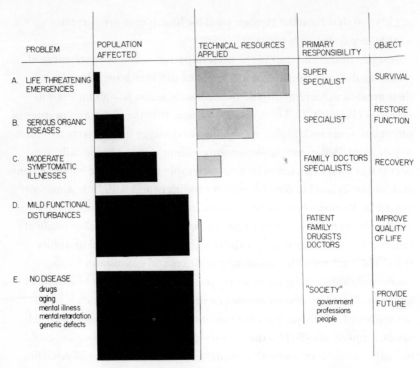

Figure 1.3 The most sophisticated technical resources, commonly operated by highly specialized personnel, are generally being utilized to extend the lives of patients with life-threatening emergencies (A). Technology is utilized to a lesser degree in efforts to restore function to the numerous patients who suffer serious organic disease (B). Moderate symptomatic illnesses affect much larger segments of the population, but their treatment involves very limited technologies (C). Mild functional disturbances (D) and health-related problems (E) interfere with the quality of life of enormous numbers of people and are generally managed ineffectually. From R. F. Rushmer, *Medical Engineering: Projections for Health Care Delivery* (New York: Academic Press, 1970), with permission of the publisher.

economics, physics, political science, chemistry, mathematics, and computer science.[4] A growing number of institutions are designed solely to investigate systematic methods for understanding man's future potentials.[5] The published literature in the field is now so extensive that it is difficult to encompass it all in a limited space.

Trend Extrapolation

In everyday life we all make decisions based on the assumption that recent trends will continue into the future. Both trivial and important decisions are made on this basis. However, this basic assumption is not as tenable in the present period of rapid change as it might have been two decades ago.

Some deficiencies of trend extrapolation revolve around the fact that the accuracy of a projection becomes progressively less reliable as it extends further and further into the future. In addition certain types of trend are much more subject to change than others. Even more important are unexpected and unpredictable changes in human values and attitudes. It would have required the highest level of genius to have accurately predicted the changes in attitude toward marriage, sex, abortion, and birth control that have occurred among the American people within the last five years. Similarly, recent changes in attitude toward the law, as expressed in violence and criminal activity, would probably not have been predicted fifteen years ago. Despite these deficiencies trend extrapolation will retain an important role. What will be needed is an increasing quantity of objective information coupled with more precisely defined criteria.

Techniques for the extrapolation of trends are becoming more sophisticated. Factor analysis can be used to identify parameters or variables that will correlate with one another to provide a multidimensional look at trends. The advent of high-speed computers now makes it possible for a very large number of interacting elements to be taken into account through the use of mathematical models of various social and economic factors.

Simulation and Modeling Methods

The human intellect has only a limited capacity to visualize the interactions of three or more variables. For example, the impact of a single factor such as population growth on energy requirements can be visualized graphically or in one's imagination, but to get a full view of the need for energy in the future one must simultaneously take into consideration a vast number of other complex, highly interrelated factors. Machine aids are obviously needed.

Simulation modeling or dynamic analysis is a technique that is being widely used today in studies of economics, social behavior, and political activities, and also in models of the economics of health, education, crime, and technological change. One interesting application of dynamic simulation and modeling is set forth in the book *Limits to Growth* by Donnela and Dennis Meadows and their colleagues.[6] In their study, Jay Forrester's world model was analyzed in terms of predictions regarding population growth, food supplies, the utilization of resources, and the technological advances that might be called upon to accommodate such changes. The results were not optimistic:

Although we have many reservations about the approximations and simplifications in the present world model, it has led us to one conclusion that appears to be justified under all the assumptions we have tested so far. The basic behavior mode of the world system is exponential growth of population and capital, followed by collapse. As we have shown in the model runs presented here, this behavior mode occurs if we assume no change in the present system or if we assume any number of technological changes in the system.

This startling conclusion has been roundly criticized by other "experts," but this has not completely suppressed the sense of insecurity the study has engendered in people in many walks of life, including the highest levels of government.

Mathematical models and computer simulations have been used extensively for the dynamic analysis of many components of the health-care delivery system. The models have varied in scope from individual laboratories to regional health-care systems and have proved quite useful in providing increased insight into their problems. The most notable contribution of this approach so far has been the identification of the *kinds* of data that must be collected if a situation is to be simulated in a meaningful way. In the case of large and complex health-care facilities in particular, the available data are seriously deficient in quantity, specificity, scope, and relevance. Moreover the greatest single deficiency, a lack of criteria for the *quality* of health care, will be hard to overcome since we have difficulty even defining health, sickness, or health care. Despite these reservations it seems safe to predict that simulation techniques have valuable contributions to make in the study of health-care systems.

Decision Trees

A sequence of key decision points can be converted into a decision tree as a graphic device for displaying the consequences of various alternatives. Such trees point up the necessary conditions required to attain long-range objectives and also indicate the points at which progress might be interrupted. Several alternatives may be available at each of the branch points, and in some cases a decision at one level may feed back to decisions at other levels to produce a more complicated picture of the process. Very large decision trees can be impressed upon computers so that scenarios and future alternatives can be generated from these basic patterns. In addition graphic and computer-generated decision trees may become key elements in initial diagnosis by paramedical personnel or by patients (see Chapter 5).

These brief descriptions do not cover all the techniques currently being employed to project future events. The most commonly used methodologies were included only to illustrate future prospects.

Examples of some of these forecasting methods applied to medicine will help to clarify the distinctions between them. Consider an example based on the following question: "What percentage of U.S. physicians will use computer diagnostic services by 1985?" (See *The Futurist* 6:24.)

1. *Intuition.* In a workshop involving physicians and computer experts and based on subjective judgment, a speaker predicts that by 1985 approximately 65% of U.S. physicians will employ computers based on increasing experimentation in automation.

2. *Trend extrapolation.* The percentage of physicians using diagnostic services increased from 4% to 27% over the past fifteen years. Continuing that trend would suggest that some 65% of physicians will employ computer diagnosis by 1985.

3. *Trend correlation.* A forecast might be based on data showing that the percentage of physicians having access to computer consultation is closely linked to three other factors: increased group practice, coverage by

insurance, and the number of physicians graduating from schools with computer instruction. Projections of these three factors have been made through 1985 and form a basis for predicting computer applications.

4. *Modeling and simulation.* Trend correlation can be extended to include integration of a complex computer model consisting of many equations representing different trends (e.g., physician work loads, specialization, consultative service, cost of computer services, etc.). Using various combinations of variables, one can draw a general picture for the year 1985.

These methods share the common deficiency of being passive and incapable of including unexpected developments, innovations, or changing values.

Group Consensus (Delphi Technique)

Wise leaders have always sought the advice and guidance of "experts." For this purpose an expert is defined as an individual whose judgment has proved better than average in anticipating likely events. The combined opinion of several experts should be more reliable than the views of a single one, but one strong personality in a group may dominate wiser heads. The Delphi Technique is one approach for combining the opinions of many experts without a face-to-face confrontation, thereby eliminating persuasion as an overriding factor. A group of possible or technological accomplishments are first described in questionnaires to a group of selected experts. They are asked to estimate the time at which these developments are most likely to occur in the future. The responses are collated, and the results of the initial inquiry are then mailed back to the same group of experts. This provides an opportunity for them to reconsider their opinion in light of the opinions of others. After a series of iterations of this process the range of dates within which the particular developments are expected to occur are presented by standard diagrams. An application of this technique is illustrated in Figure 1.4, derived from a study of developments in medicine by A. Douglas Bender and his colleagues.[7] A geometrical figure, shaped roughly like a hip-roofed building with a peak near the center, is constructed to illustrate the range of projected dates for the anticipated accomplishment. The highest point of the figure indicates the most frequent (median) estimate. The highest level of confidence is

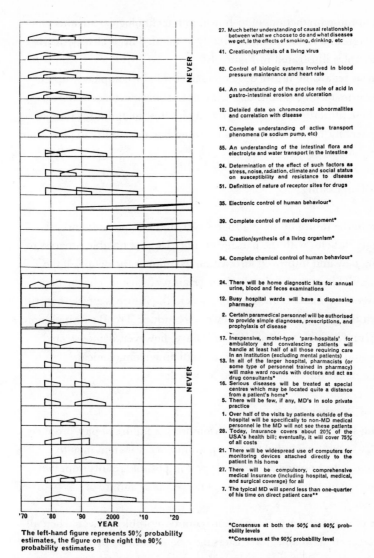

27. Much better understanding of causal relationship between what we choose to do and what diseases we get, ie the effects of smoking, drinking. etc

41. Creation/synthesis of a living virus

62. Control of biologic systems involved in blood pressure maintenance and heart rate

64. An understanding of the precise role of acid in gastro-intestinal erosion and ulceration

12. Detailed data on chromosomal abnormalities and correlation with disease

17. Complete understanding of active transport phenomena (ie sodium pump, etc)

65. An understanding of the intestinal flora and electrolyte and water transport in the intestine

24. Determination of the effect of such factors as stress, noise, radiation, climate and social status on susceptibility and resistance to disease

51. Definition of nature of receptor sites for drugs

35. Electronic control of human behaviour*

39. Complete control of mental development*

43. Creation/synthesis of a living organism*

34. Complete chemical control of human behaviour*

24. There will be home diagnostic kits for annual urine, blood and feces examinations

12. Busy hospital wards will have a dispensing pharmacy

2. Certain paramedical personnel will be authorised to provide simple diagnoses, prescriptions, and prophylaxis of disease

17. Inexpensive, motel-type 'para-hospitals' for ambulatory and convalescing patients will handle at least half of all those requiring care in an institution (excluding mental patients)

13. In all of the larger hospital, pharmacists (or some type of personnel trained in pharmacy) will make ward rounds with doctors and act as drug consultants*

16. Serious diseases will be treated at special centres which may be located quite a distance from a patient's home*

5. There will be few, if any, MD's in solo private practice

1. Over half of the visits by patients outside of the hospital will be specifically to non-MD medical personnel ie the MD will not see these patients

28. Today, insurance covers about 20% of the USA's health bill; eventually, it will cover 75% of all costs

21. There will be widespread use of computers for monitoring devices attached directly to the patient in his home

27. There will be compulsory, comprehensive medical insurance (including hospital, medical, and surgical coverage) for all

7. The typical MD will spend less than one-quarter of his time on direct patient care**

'70   '80   '90   2000   '10   '20
YEAR

The left-hand figure represents 50% probability estimates, the figure on the right the 90% probability estimates

*Consensus at both the 50% and 90% probability levels

**Consensus at the 90% probability level

Figure 1.4 A consensus of expert opinion regarding the likelihood of various future developments in medicine as obtained by the Delphi Technique. The times at which the developments listed on the right will reach fruition are indicated at the 50% and 90% probability levels by geometrical figures spanning the next fifty-odd years. The upper and lower 25% of the estimates are eliminated, producing the blunted extremes. The peak of each geometrical figure indicates the median value. These are representative examples from a larger study by A. Douglas Bender and coworkers.[7]

obtained in those predictions of technical and technological advances for which background information is already at hand. This is clearly the case in the examples illustrated in Figure 1.4.

Consensus regarding future developments could be completely upset by new discoveries or innovations that have not yet been even considered. Despite these limitations there is a growing interest in and utilization of consensus techniques of various sorts to strengthen our ability to plan more effectively for the future.

Limits to Forecasting

Peering into the future becomes progressively more important and yet increasingly difficult with the passage of time. Despite notable progress in developing new and improved forecasting techniques the details of the future are still obscured by clouds of uncertainty. Marking out the best path between the many immediate barriers to the future is a task that still defies both the traditional and the newer techniques. Trend extrapolation, modeling, and group consensus (Delphi) have, however, demonstrated reliability and improved consistency in predicting technological developments on the basis of current knowledge.

Hazards of Prophecy

Examining some of the underlying reasons for the failure of past prophets, Arthur C. Clarke[8] concluded that the inability of competent men to predict what is technologically possible and impossible results from two main factors, which he terms "failure of nerve" and "failure of imagination."

Failure of nerve seems to be the more common problem. Even when all relevant facts are available, forecasters may be so blinded by imagined dangers or so set in their present ways that they deny the conclusion to which the facts seem inevitably to lead. For example, when the first locomotives were being contemplated, dire predictions were often voiced that suffocation would threaten anyone traveling faster than 30 miles an hour, and more recently the possibility of breaking the sound barrier was denied because of the putative ill effects of supersonic flight. Edison opposed the introduction of alternating current, steadfastly insisting that direct current was the only sensible way to transmit electrical power. And failure of nerve can also be held responsible for the fact that so many of the world's leading authorities disclaimed any suggestion that human flight might be possible, much less the successful transmission of humans to the moon.

Clarke concluded that anything theoretically possible will be achieved in practice *if it is desired enough.* To avoid the failure of nerve that has plagued man's past history it is necessary to retain confidence in the ingenuity of mankind. It is harder to get around failure of imagination, since no one can predict a development that has not yet been conceived. On all sides we see classes of inventions that could easily have been understood or predicted by the great thinkers of the past as intuitive possibilities. Benjamin Franklin, Leonardo da Vinci, and Archimedes would not have been startled by a steam engine or a helicopter. They would have been utterly amazed at the reality of a television set, a computer, or a nuclear reactor.

The contrast between predictable developments and those that cannot be anticipated is suggested by the representative lists in Table 1.1. There are many modern accomplishments that would have been inconceivable in 1900. Looking ahead, it is surprisingly difficult to clearly distinguish possible future developments from the "utterly impossible."

Table 1.1

The Expected	The Unexpected
automobiles	x-rays
flying machines	nuclear energy
steam engines	radio, television
submarines	electronics
spaceships	photography
telephones	sound recording
robots	quantum mechanics
death rays	relativity
transmutation	transistors
artificial life	masers, lasers
levitation	superconductors, superfluids
telepathy	atomic clocks, the Mössbauer effect
	determining the composition of celestial bodies
	dating the past (carbon 14, etc.)
	detecting invisible planets
	the ionosphere, Van Allen belts

After Arthur C. Clarke.[8]

Unpredicted Innovations

The most important obstacle to accurate prediction of the future is, then, the fact that one cannot fully anticipate those revolutionary discoveries that change the course of history in fundamental ways. For example, totally accidental observations have resulted in such fundamental discoveries as x-rays, penicillin, and electricity. To make the assumption that our future is totally dependent upon our current level of knowledge without considering the possibility of totally new and revolutionary discoveries is a serious failure of imagination. A backward look provides ample assurance that new discoveries will be made with even greater frequency in the future.

Even more significant is the prospect that the conversion of new discoveries into useful commercial devices and innovations will continue to occur with shorter and shorter time lags. John McHale[9] has presented a graphic representation of the progressive shortening of the time elapsing between discoveries and applications in the physical sciences (Figure 1.5). The interval between the discovery of principles and the utilization of photography was 112 years, while the telephone and electric motor required 56 and 65 years respectively. A progressive shortening of the lag times for the conversion of basic discoveries into useful applications has occurred with radio, x-rays, radar, and television. Huge amounts of talent and resources were focused on the development of the atomic bomb only six years after nuclear fission was demonstrated, and, more recently, transistors were commercially produced some three years after their first experimental demonstration and have greatly influenced the entire electronics industry.

The explosive expansion of scientific information is still occurring in myriad basic and applied research-and-development laboratories. The rapid conversion of new knowledge into new technology is as clearly evident in medicine as in other segments of our society. Our long-range plans must not neglect the probability that technological advances, currently beyond our power to foresee, may greatly simplify and improve the various processes involved in data acquisition, information management, and the diagnosis, therapy, monitoring, and management of acute and chronic illnesses. For these reasons the passive projection of coming

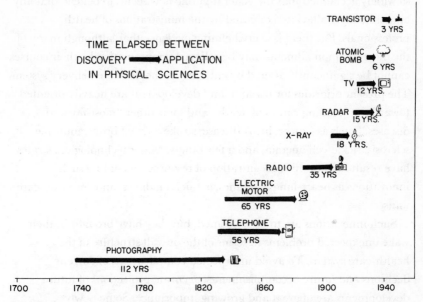

TIME ELAPSED BETWEEN
DISCOVERY ➡ APPLICATION
IN PHYSICAL SCIENCES

TRANSISTOR ➡ 3 YRS

ATOMIC
BOMB ➡ 6 YRS

TV ➡ 12 YRS.

RADAR ➡ 15 YRS.

X-RAY ➡ 18 YRS.

RADIO ➡ 35 YRS

ELECTRIC
MOTOR
65 YRS

TELEPHONE
56 YRS

PHOTOGRAPHY
112 YRS

| 1700 | 1740 | 1780 | 1820 | 1860 | 1900 | 1940 |

Figure 1.5 Projecting future possibilities is complicated by the accelerating transition of new discoveries into practical applications. The lag time from demonstrated feasibility to commercial production has been reduced from more than one hundred years for photography to less than three years for transistors. Redrawn from John McHale's *World Facts and Trends*.[9]

events from current trends limits the effectiveness of long-range planning.

Summary

During the past few decades amazing progress has been made in the application of scientific medicine and surgery to the diagnosis and effective therapy of an expanding array of diseases and disabilities. During this same period, however, the general public has demonstrated an increasing disenchantment with the present health-care delivery system.

Major causes of public criticism can be traced to exaggerated expectations and to the loss of personal support and individual concern that has accompanied specialization. Indeed the medical triumphs and technical spectaculars of the past few decades have been so impressive and so widely acclaimed that the general public now seems to believe that any ailment can be alleviated or cured by the ministrations of health professionals. But there is overwhelming evidence that, although many of the most common ailments may be relieved symptomatically, their courses cannot be significantly altered by entering the health-care delivery system. The present priorities for research and development are heavily oriented toward the "leading causes of death" and some other "most-favored diseases," such as cancer, heart disease, stroke, cystic fibrosis, multiple sclerosis, sickle-cell anemia, and a few others. Major technological strides have resulted from this concentration of resources, including such innovations as heart-lung machines, artificial kidneys, and coronary-care units.

Such innovations are to be welcomed, but they have brought in their wake unexpected problems in terms of the overall structure of the health-care system. To avoid unexpected complications of current decisions and future accomplishments, accurate projections of future developments are of great and growing importance. Some newly developed techniques of future forecasting are under intensive study, including trend extrapolation, model simulation, and group-census techniques.

These approaches help to provide perspective, but there are many barriers to accurate prophecy. Failure of nerve can blind us to the drift of facts, and failure of imagination can cause us to miss the unexpected developments that so often prove to be of fundamental importance. In addition, the rate of accumulation of knowledge and of scientific progress always tends to exceed expectations. Finally, present methods of prediction are totally incapable of predicting major shifts in social, economic, and political attitudes. A more effective approach to long-range planning is sorely needed for future health-care delivery. One possibility is the concept of *creating desirable futures*, which will be presented in the next chapter.

References

1. George A. Silver. 1970. American medicine: Technology outruns social usefulness. *Bull. N.Y. Acad. Med.* 46:148–160.
2. Anne R. Somers. 1971. *Health Care in Transition: Directions for the Future.* Chicago: Hospital Research and Educational Trust.
3. Irving Page. 1967. Yesterday, today and tomorrow. *J. Am. Med. Assoc.* 201:256–259.

4. John McHale. 1970. A survey of futures research in the United States. *The Futurist* 4:200–204.

5. Theodore J. Gordon. 1972. Current methods of futures research. In *The Futurists,* ed., Alvin Toffler. New York: Random House.

6. Donella H. Meadows, Dennis L. Meadows, Jørgen Randers, and William W. Behrens III. 1972. *Limits to Growth.* New York: Universe Books.

7. A. Douglas Bender, Alvin E. Strack, George W. Elbright, and George von Hanualter. 1969. Delphic study examines developments in medicine. *Futures* 1:289–303.

8. Arthur C. Clarke. 1972. Hazards of prophecy. In *The Futurists,* ed., Alvin Toffler. New York: Random House.

9. John McHale. 1972. *World Facts and Trends.* 2nd ed. New York: Macmillan.

2
Creating Desirable Futures for Health Care

The forecasting of future events by the methods described in Chapter 1 is intended to facilitate the making of plans, policies, and decisions on a more rational basis than mere intuition. Unfortunately there are always powerful deterrents to the development of plans or programs to be pursued in the immediate future. All the vested interests, controversial issues, and polarization of attitudes concerning "the next step" impede initial action toward improvement. It is frequently easier to obtain agreement regarding what ought to be accomplished ten or twenty years in the future than to obtain an effective consensus regarding what needs to be done next week or next year. Thus it is not surprising that the concept of identifying long-range goals for desirable futures is attracting a great deal of favorable attention among organizations, institutions, states, and regions.

The creation of desirable futures depends upon the careful selection and concise definition of long-range goals using opinions solicited from widely diversified sources (Figure 2.1). These long-range goals then serve as the basis for setting and maintaining courses of action, fundamental policies, and sequential decisions all directed toward common and visible objectives over a long period of time. To accommodate to changes that may intervene with the passage of time, the goals must be periodically reassessed and modified.

Each goal can be interpreted in terms of its identifiable requirements, including the many different options by which essential needs can be met. The different options are often mutually compatible, however, so that several may be employed simultaneously with each one contributing to the total effect while providing mutual support for other parallel efforts. A prime characteristic of this basic approach is that many different approaches can be developed concurrently to facilitate progress toward identifiable objectives.

Conversion of Objections into Objectives for Long-Range Planning

A simple way to begin identifying long-range goals is to assemble the most prominent criticisms or objections from as wide a variety of reliable sources

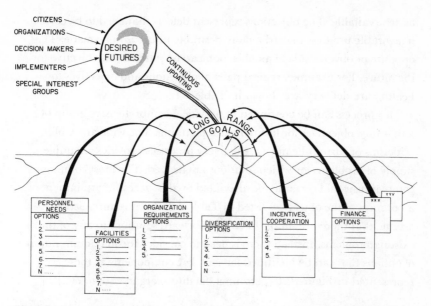

Figure 2.1 A potentially powerful approach to the future involves the clear and concise definition of long-range goals (ten to twenty years ahead) viewed as desirable futures, preferably based on maximal input from many different sources. The ultimate shape of these goals can be specified in terms of personnel needs, facilities, organizational requirements, etc., and a variety of options can be specified for meeting these needs. Positive efforts can then be directed toward realizing such options whenever decisions must be made in the course of time. A variety of sample options is presented in the text to elucidate the principles involved.

Table 2.1

Objection	Objective
Unavailable nights or weekends	Available any time, day or night
Physician-centered	Patient-centered
Impersonal	Warm and sympathetic
Disease-oriented	Individual-oriented
Inefficient	Efficient
Excessively expensive	Reasonably priced

as are available. The objections represent defects that need to be corrected if favorable progress toward a more desirable future is to be made. The opposite or obverse side of an objection can be stated as an objective for the future. For example, typical pairs of objections and objectives for health-care delivery are shown in Table 2.1.

This process can be continued to provide a comprehensive group of long-range objectives for future health planning. The wide array of criticisms of current health-care delivery processes provides an ample supply of problems for which solutions are desired. The most common complaints would certainly be alleviated by the successful attainment of all or most of the objectives listed in Table 2.2. But it is unrealistic to assume that there are simple or straightforward solutions to any of the existing problems. Instead there is need to consider the maximum number of options that can be identified for such key components as those represented in Figure 2.1 (personnel, facilities, organization, etc.).

Identifying Objections, Objectives, and Opportunities

A number of perceptive analyses of the many and varied problems of health care have been published in the past few years.[1,2,3,4] A common approach revolves around problems related to (1) health personnel, (2) patients, (3) hospitals, (4) organization, and (5) costs. Certain issues recur

Table 2.2
Sample Objectives for Improving Health-Care Delivery

1. Ready access, convenience, and dependability
2. Availability any time, any place
3. Appropriate and effective action
4. Assurance of quality and thoroughness
5. Continuity and consistency
6. Warm and sympathetic relationships
7. Concern for the whole patient
8. Understanding of the person, his family, and environment
9. Patient-centered: patient consulted and informed
10. Organization of efforts for convenience and welfare of the patient
11. Improved geographic distribution
12. Equitable socioeconomic distribution
13. Comprehensive and well-organized
14. Integrated and efficient
15. Reasonable cost

with sufficient regularity that they probably reflect a degree of consensus regarding key defects or deficiencies. Far less unanimity can be discovered among the proposed corrective measures. Identification and definition of the major defects in the system are clearly necessary first steps toward reasonable and desirable approaches.

Shortage of Physicians?

The public gains a general impression that there is a shortage of physicians and facilities whenever a sick patient cannot gain prompt access to effective care when he needs it and is able and prepared to pay for it.[2] When a patient wishes to consult with his physician and must wait days or even weeks for an appointment, he is convinced that there are insufficient doctors to fill his needs. Increasingly, persons who develop symptoms of illness at night or on weekends cannot locate an available physician. They flock to the emergency rooms of hospitals, clogging these facilities to the point that real emergencies are neglected. Examples of patients who are acutely ill and cannot locate available medical help have solidified the impression that a major shortage of physicians exists. As a result additional incentives have been introduced by the federal government to increase the sizes of medical classes so that more doctors can be trained. A rapid expansion in the number of physicians will not, however, solve the complex problems that confront the health-care delivery system.

The Physician-Centered System

Current personnel shortages result in part from the traditional patient-doctor relationship. Richard Magraw,[3] in discussing this relationship, has stressed the concept of a "psychology of illness" that is responsible for an element of trust being necessary if the patient is to obtain maximum benefit from medical care and if the painful, frightening, and discouraging effects of illness are to be assuaged.

Extensive dependence by both patients and physicians on this complicated and intangible relationship is directly responsible for one major source of economic inefficiency, namely the fact that, although the physician is by far the highest paid member of the health team, he is personally involved in time-consuming routines during each successive step of management. This utter dependence of all concerned on the physician was desirable and effective when he functioned as a lone agent without the trappings and complexity of modern medicine. As the leader of a diverse health-care team, however, this unique axial position breeds enormous inefficiencies and costs. Although high costs are the most tangible stress on the health-care delivery system, the chief complaints by consumers are more commonly directed at deficiencies of a more personal sort. Sick people feel betrayed and abandoned by a profession that formerly enjoyed a high position of respect and prestige as being selfless, sympathetic, and available. Indeed today's highly specialized physicians seem to pay more attention to the disease than to the patient as a person.

Availability of Health Care When and Where It Is Needed

When the medical profession abandoned the concept of being available at the convenience of the patient, it failed to make other provisions for this requirement. The responsibility was delegated to no one else, leaving an unfulfilled obligation (see Chapters 6 and 7).

The long tradition of doctors being freely available day or night and willing to make house calls was disrupted and largely discarded during World War II, when a large proportion of the physicians in both military and civilian life discovered that it was possible and more efficient to practice medicine in offices or hospitals. They found that they could see more patients, diagnose and treat illnesses more efficiently, and live a much more pleasant and productive life by imposing more standard working hours. Many other factors mitigated against the retention of the long-standing rapport between "family" doctors and their patients. The greatly increased mobility of the American family, the reduction in the cohesiveness of the family unit, the trend toward medical specialization, and the recognized lack of an adequate number of family physicians, all helped to disrupt the traditional doctor-patient relationship. There are simply not enough general practitioners available to make house calls a practical method of health delivery, and highly trained medical and surgical specialists are neither prepared nor equipped to serve in the role of warm and patient family counselors, particularly when they function in a hospital setting. The sound advice and guidance that the public needs in its pursuit of improved health are simply not being adequately provided by the medical profession as currently constituted.

It thus appears necessary to consider delegating the responsibility for health promotion, counseling, and continuity to specially trained members of *primary-care teams* (see Chapter 7). This is but one example of an apparent health-personnel shortage *outside* the ranks of highly trained physicians and of the need for competent and trained people capable of serving vital functions within the organizational framework of modern medicine. Indeed, while the number of physicians in active practice has grown at about the same rate as the general population,[5] the number of professional nurses, nonprofessional nurses, and medical auxiliary personnel (radiologists and clinical-laboratory personnel) has increased at three times that rate. Enormous growth has also occurred in other categories of paraprofessional and supportive personnel, including pharmacists, dieticians, clinical psychologists, rehabilitation counselors, special technicians, and various kinds of therapists (occupational, physical, speech, hearing, inhalation, etc.). It is thus extremely important to view the problem of personnel shortages in terms of the entire health-care community, including professionals, paraprofessionals, and the support personnel needed for the essential functions of health-care delivery. The sources of dissatisfaction mentioned above can be more readily dispelled under ideal conditions by the provision of:

1. prompt and easy access to appropriate health-care personnel;
2. increased time available for direct contact between the patient and the appropriate member(s) of the health-care team;
3. extended services that are readily available to anyone, at any time and place, in amounts and of a kind appropriate for the patient's needs;
4. delivery of health care organized for the convenience of the patient with an optimal ratio of cost to benefit (see Chapter 3).

Impersonalization

It is generally agreed that much of the personal involvement and sympathy that so characterized the "old-fashioned family doctor" is missing in many settings today. There is no reason, however, why these qualities could not be shared by other members of the health-care team if their responsibility were self-limited and if adequate training and supervision were to assure necessary competence. On this basis an objective for the future might be individualization of care through more effective utilization of an increasingly diverse health-care team.

Effective Utilization

Patients who must wait hours after the appointed time to see their physician become justifiably annoyed. Rashi Fein[2] has noted a national survey of pediatricians in which 40% of those responding complained that they were "too busy." Studies conducted on the activities of pediatricians engaged in active practice, however, revealed that 50% of the working day was spent with healthy children and 22% with children having minor respiratory illnesses.[6] Only about 10% of a pediatrician's time may be devoted to the management of the type and severity of illness and dysfunction for which he has spent years and thousands of dollars being trained. Recognition that a very large portion of a pediatrician's activities can be effectively handled without the M.D. degree has stimulated the development of training programs for nurse practitioners,[7] physician's assistants, and other medical paraprofessionals.

Pediatrics is a rather extreme example, but many other types of physicians dissipate their time in unrewarding routines that can be done better by other trained members of the team. There are many opportunities to insure the effective utilization of the physician's time, to broaden professional opportunities, and to overcome some of the organizational deficiencies of medical practice that are discussed in more detail below and in subsequent chapters.

Maldistribution of Physicians and Facilities

Considering only the total number of physicians (and allied health personnel) may give a seriously distorted picture of the real situation because the *distribution* of medical personnel in cities, towns, and rural areas bears little relationship to either the population or the need. Physicians living in wealthy suburban areas near large cities find life extremely pleasant, professional contacts and facilities convenient, and patients relatively healthy, well-nourished, and able to pay. For these reasons physicians tend to congregate in and near large urban centers in numbers amounting to a major surplus. For example, New York City contains about 4% of the population of the United States, but 9% of the physicians are located there.[8] Imagine, nearly one doctor in every ten in this country lives in a very small area in and around Manhattan Island, yet its ghettos contain thousands of people lacking even minimal care.

The number of physicians is totally inadequate in both the centers of major cities and the more remote rural areas because the depression of living conditions and incomes in these areas are powerful disincentives to physicians. Incentives that might encourage physicians to settle in such locations have proved largely ineffectual. One current alternative is to train paraprofessionals to help relieve the heavy work loads of rural and center-city physicians. There is really no prospect of ever providing health-care personnel and facilities in the quantity and quality required to cover all the needs of residents of these areas; but this would not be necessary if we would more effectively utilize our sophisticated communications network and transportation capabilities to transmit information from patients to medical centers and to convey patients to the appropriate facilities for the treatment of their illnesses.

The Soaring Costs of Health-Care Delivery

The most obvious symptom of dysfunction of the health-care system is the skyrocketing of costs. Although the prices of many goods and services have been increasing rather steadily in recent years, the upward spiral of medical expenditures has outstripped all others (Figure 2.2). In the seventeen years between 1955 and 1972 total expenditures climbed from about $17 billion to some $83 billion, and it is currently anticipated that the annual expenditure for health will rise well above $100 billion. Indeed, if one includes the costs of worktime lost because of illness and the money expended for prevention, rehabilitation, and research, the annual financial impact greatly exceeds $100 billion today. The largest total increase has been in private funds, which includes insurance, but the largest percentage increase has been in federal support, particularly for the Medicare and Medicaid programs. The problems confronting senior citizens can be emphasized by noting that the average annual cost per person for medical care increases from $140 for individuals below age 19 to $323 for those between 20 and 65, to a whopping $851 for those past 65, who are usually far from affluent.

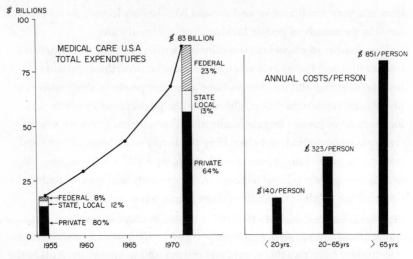

Figure 2.2 The soaring cost of medical care between 1955 and 1972 includes a growing contribution by federal and state governments, but these sources still total less than half of the $83 billion national health bill (left). The highest costs for health care are imposed on the older population, many of whom find themselves without the resources to pay (right).

Unfortunately the steeply rising costs have not been accompanied by a corresponding improvement in either the quantity or quality of health care. Despite the enormous expenditures for health care and health maintenance during the past fifty years the life expectancy of the average man 40 years old has been increased by only about two years. Meanwhile the death rates of teenagers, young adults, and the younger middle-aged have substantially increased (due more, it must be noted, to changing life styles than to the mechanisms of health-care delivery). There is thus no clear relationship between the current expenditures for health care and any overall improvement in the health status of the citizenry.[4] A major effort must be expended to utilize more effectively the personnel and services that are presently available and to attempt to curtail costs by more attention to cost-effectiveness and the ratio of cost to benefit (see Chapter 3). An essential step is to evaluate critically some of the causes of these steadily climbing costs.[9,10,11]

Some Factors Contributing to Increasing Physicians' Fees and Charges
In the American economy doctors and their representatives have insisted
on fees for service, and rising demand has produced correspondingly
higher incomes. But physicians react to the law of supply and demand
differently from other groups in that an increased demand for health care
produces increased service through longer hours and more visits per hour.
Even if the value of each visit diminishes, the physician's income increases
greatly even though the fee for each visit increases only gradually.

To some extent the rise in doctors' incomes may be associated with
increased productivity. In the early postwar period prices in general rose
rapidly, while physician fees increased at a much slower rate. This
indicates that physicians passed on the gains of rising productivity to the
patient. However, this trend has not been evident in the 1970s, and total
costs have thus risen more sharply. Furthermore the increased productivity
may be due to improved facilities and therapeutic effectiveness, concealing
to some extent the deterioration of service from packed appointments,
hurried visits, and decreased availability.

The causes and consequences of thoroughness
A common criterion for the quality of a physician's service is thoroughness.
Generally accepted standards calling for a comprehensive search for
disease and disability are enforced by the patient, by the patient's family,
by medical colleagues, and by the community in general. From his earliest
training in medical school a physician is roundly criticized if he misses a
diagnosis or has a discouraging therapeutic result because he has failed to
take advantage of opportunities to test or treat. He is rarely subject to
criticism for having excessive zeal in his testing or retesting, examination
or reexamination, prolonged therapy or hospital stays and follow-up.
Threats of lawsuits for malpractice are multiplying rapidly, and the only
real protection against exorbitant judgments in such suits is to have
covered all eventualities. (In 1971 the number of malpractice suits reached
levels between 7,000 and 10,000.) Thus, given that the cost of the extra
tests or examinations is borne by the patient or his insurance, the
physician has little to gain and much to lose by showing restraint in the
use of hospital facilities or in the number and frequency of tests.

The cost of reassurance

A very large percentage of persons visiting physicians have minor ailments or symptoms that are not functionally significant. The physician is reluctant to dismiss these symptoms and reassure the patient unless he has become quite convinced that he is not overlooking something more serious. Similarly the patient is likely to be unconvinced or dissatisfied by a physician's assurance that he need not worry unless he has received a fairly extensive examination. Thus both the patient and the physician frequently require reassurance through comprehensive examinations even in the absence of significant dysfunction. Since the incidence of minor complaints is so very high, the overall cost of this kind of reassurance is astronomical. The development of highly organized and inexpensive multiphasic screening facilities may ultimately have great value in reducing the cost of uncertainty and the expenditures for reassurance, and allied health personnel may also play a greater role in supplementing this function (see Chapter 5).

The requirement for thoroughness evolved in an age when available tests were few and cheap. At that time comprehensive examinations merely provided a longer personal contact between the physician and his patient. The beneficial result of more careful examination and prolonged deliberation were obvious. However, unrestrained thoroughness and a comprehensive approach to medical care is at present imposing an enormous drain on the resources of the medical community. The common practice of ordering a large variety of complex and expensive tests, repeated at frequent intervals, is extremely costly and has not been critically examined to determine the extent to which it actually improves health care. When a patient is referred to another physician, the consultant frequently repeats already performed tests and adds more. Only the most secure and self-confident physician can muster the courage to be content with minimal or optimal diagnostic tests. Competent physicians could conserve funds without jeopardy to the patient, but they would do so at the risk of criticism or legal liability in malpractice suits.

The Rising Costs of Hospitalization

The most challenging problem in the health-care delivery system is the role of the modern hospital. Cost is one obvious and important aspect of this complex problem. From 1940 to 1961 daily charges increased by some 380%,[9] while the costs of more specialized auxiliary services underwent comparable increases. There is no way of judging whether this increased cost is justified in terms of increased value received because there is no generally accepted yardstick for the product (see Chapter 3).

In all this complex organizational framework there exists no implicit mechanism or pressure to restrain costs or to introduce economy in the care of hospitalized patients. The physician charges fees that are independent of the unit costs of the hospital stay or the special tests and services ordered. The hospital makes charges that are designed to defray expenses no matter how large they may be. This form of "cost-plus" economics, which has proven extremely costly in military contracts, has also contributed significantly to the rapidly spiraling costs of patient care. In general hospital administrators like to preserve high rates of cash flow, with less attention to economy. Indeed an increase in productivity or efficiency that would cause empty beds or reduce the use of services would tend to further imbalance the precarious state of the hospital.

An important element in rising costs is lack of efficiency in the utilization of personnel. A generally accepted principle of sound management is to assign tasks to the person with the least amount of training qualified to perform the job. In hospitals, however, one often finds highly trained individuals performing routine or menial chores. In the past, when some need for additional service has arisen, the standard response has been to add more personnel. Expanded numbers of health-care personnel, coupled with recent trends toward rapidly rising wages, are key elements in the soaring costs of hospitalization.

Too many hospital beds
Excess costs of hospitalization are compounded by the fact that we have so many beds that substantial numbers lie empty. On an average day last year about 318,000 hospital beds, one out of five, were empty across the United States. Obviously some hospitals are full and have waiting lists, but there are several thousand empty hospital beds in New York City alone, and six cities are reported to have 4,000 beds more than they need. The costs of hospitalization are greatly increased when the occupancy rates diminish. This "excessive" construction of hospitals has been due in part to

rather indiscriminate federal support through "Hill-Burton" funds (see Chapter 6).

The prevailing pattern of ownership and control of health facilities is the voluntary nonprofit hospital. Hospitals are granted nonprofit status to avoid the pressures for economy that are found in competitive profit-making enterprises. They are not required by any pressure to achieve economies or to accomplish high levels of efficiency. In fact they may be roundly criticized if they are caught cutting corners. The controlling motivation in hospital design is to be safe rather than sorry; extra capabilities and stand-by facilities are built and maintained in order to meet *any possible* problem, rather than to accommodate only the probable requirements of a particular clientele.

This brief review of some factors contributing to the current health-care "crisis" was designed to indicate a constructive approach to the defects. More extensive discussion of these problems can be found in numerous other publications.[1,2,3,4] A more detailed consideration of options that should be considered as means to overcome deficiencies in personnel, facilities, and organizational relationships are presented in subsequent chapters, particularly 5–8.

Broadened Definitions of Health

Any comprehensive consideration of sickness and disability demands a definition of health. Most people regard health as the absence of disease, but dysfunction and disability are inevitable components of human life, so that this definition implies an unattainable ideal. Moreover the concept that health is the absence of organic pathology ignores psychosomatic disturbances and the deleterious effects of an unfavorable environment. But with growing experience it is becoming more evident that the incidence of the signs and symptoms of disease is greater in those individuals living in undesirable environments or exposed to socio-economic pressures. Thus we might usefully regard health as freedom from disease, dysfunction, and disability insofar as they interfere with the functioning of a human being in his particular environment. On this basis it seems desirable to greatly broaden our consideration of health to include physical, social, and psychological well-being.

Major obstacles to the development of universal and equal access to health and health care lie outside the sphere of influence of the health professions. Current socioeconomic conditions in our society segregate and sequester whole groups of individuals that have a high incidence of physical and emotional disability. A consideration of long-range goals for health cannot afford to neglect such a significant portion of our population.

Socioeconomic Disability: A Contributing Factor in Illness
The traditional American concept of the course of life begins with a period of extended education. This "tooling-up period" is intended to prepare people for a productive life, envisioned as a series of upward steps in accomplishment, competence, security, and rewards terminating in retirement on an income adequate to provide a comfortable period of obsolescence (see Figure 2.3A). This could be regarded as the standard American dream. Unfortunately not everyone has experiences consistent with this dream. Substantial numbers of individuals are diverted from the mainstream of American life through one-way trapdoors into a wide variety of storage bins, slots, or warehouses (Figure 2.3B). Included among these sequestered people are those individuals who drop out, either during their educational period or afterwards, prisoners, the mentally ill, the chronically ill, and the retarded. Senior citizens in retirement who were unable to put aside enough money during their productive periods to last them through their period of retirement may also find themselves in this undesirable situation. Those who drift away from the mainstream of society and fall into these categories find it difficult to recover without outside help.

People who deviate from the mainstream because of accident, necessity, or intention may be institutionalized, alienated, or disadvantaged, and the incidence of disease and disability is very high among their ranks. Susceptibility to infections such as pneumonia and tuberculosis is significantly greater among individuals living in undesirable circumstances and under psychosocial stress. Overuse and abuse of drugs are clearly as significant a cause of disability as are peptic ulcers or hypertension. The health professions cannot afford to focus their attention only on those elements of illness that are the results of organic pathological

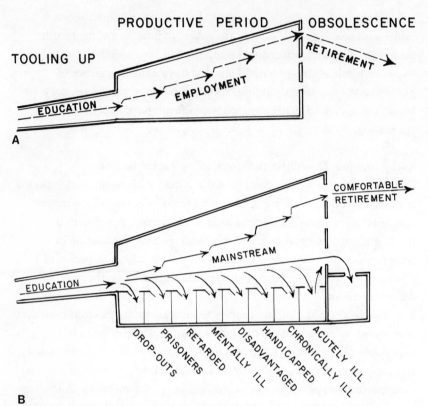

Figure 2.3 One traditional view of a lifetime begins with a period of education leading to a productive period of employment, during which sufficient resources are accumulated to permit a comfortable and pleasant period of retirement (A). In reality large portions of the population are diverted from the mainstream of life and are entrapped, estranged, or institutionalized (B). In general people who are diverted from the mainstream have great difficulty returning and usually require help. (Acute illness is a major exception to this rule.) A very high incidence of health and socioeconomic problems characterizes those diverted, isolated, or sequestered from the mainstream. Based on diagrams devised by Hewitt Crane of Stanford Research Institute.

processes and ignore the equally serious and painful dysfunctions that
result from psychological, social, or even economic pressures. The
significance of this broadened definition of health will be apparent in
many different aspects of the subsequent discussion as we approach the
requirements for the provision of adequate health care to various age
groups and segments of our society.

Common Ailments at Different Ages

The principal forms of illness that affect people at different stages in life
are indicated in Figure 2.4. The relative contributions to the family and
society are qualitatively indicated on the vertical scale. In agricultural
societies children are economic necessities. In industrialized societies,
however, young people contribute little to their family's economic
well-being and have little basis for feeling needed or useful. They
constitute a very significant drain on the family, which becomes extended

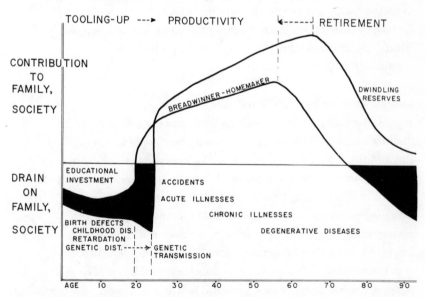

Figure 2.4 The life of an average individual is characterized by several different stages, each
having a decidedly different distribution of most common ailments. The first two decades are
dominated by the common childhood diseases. During the early productive period accidents
and acute illnesses are most common, while chronic and degenerative diseases predominate
at more advanced years. The social and economic aspects of the most common ailments in
these various age groups are rarely considered in the allocation of health resources.

if the educational process is prolonged. This initial stage of life is a period of investment in the individual leading, hopefully, toward a productive period of life.

The duration of the productive period is progressively diminishing as education is being prolonged and retirement is more frequently begun at an earlier age. For example, progressively larger numbers of workers are retiring from the production industries at 60 or even 55 years of age. This prolongs the postproductive period of retirement during which the individual lives on accumulated resources of his own, of society, or of his children. With inflation, taxes, and increased longevity the happy, tranquil years of retirement have been replaced for many by isolation from family, financial insecurity, and progressive deterioration of health.

The major current emphasis of both medical research and medical practice is the management of illnesses that predominate among older segments of the population under the assumption that the increased life expectancy will also extend the period of pleasant retirement. All too frequently these efforts inadvertently prolong periods of loneliness, frustration, and suffering. If we are going to prolong life, we must also sustain and improve its quality.

Categories of Disease and Disability

In most medical discussions malfunctions, ailments, diseases, and disabilities are lumped together as though they could be managed as a single entity. The diversity of types and severity of illness is inconsistent with this view. In the past individual citizens were obliged to accept full responsibility for most, if not all, of their ills. Now the government is assuming ever-increasing responsibility for many areas of health management. A reasonable approach to this complicated problem requires improved categorization of the various types of illness and broader consensus regarding who is to be responsible for each type. For this purpose various categories are proposed in Table 2.3 under new labels that are designed to convey the essence of the definitions wherever possible. Some of these terms may sound unfamiliar, trite, or facetious at first. They are certainly unscientific in origin. Of greater significance is the intent to provide readily recognizable terms that convey unique and specific meanings, unencumbered by previous usage where possible.

Table 2.3
Categories of Disease and Disability

	Characterization
1. Sui-sickness	A self-induced increase in hazard or risk through patient volition or indulgence (e.g., driving while drunk, smoking with chronic bronchitis, drug and alcohol abuse, skiing, mountaineering, overeating).
2. Mini-mal	A functional disturbance that interferes with the quality of life but does not produce disability (e.g., conditions commonly mentioned in mass-media advertising, such as constipation, headaches, visual disturbances, hearing losses, insomnia, skin lesions, hay fever, hyperactivity).
3. Common ill	A self-limited common illness that rarely if ever has lasting effects or complications (e.g., head colds, "flu," diarrhea, dysmenorrhea).
4. Midi-mal	An illness of moderate severity and relatively ineffective therapy; inconsequential but may produce complications or lasting effects sufficiently often to warrant medical evaluation.
5. Mendi-mal	A moderate to severe disease or disability for which therapy is directly effective (e.g., infection by organisms susceptible to antibodies, vitamin or dietary deficiencies, hormonal deficiences, peptic ulcers, hypertension).
6. Eradic-ailment	A dysfunction or disability whose cause can be eliminated through medical or surgical therapy by removing, repairing, or replacing the ailing function or part.
7. Maxi-mal	An acute threat to life and health of such severity and immediacy as to require the prompt and concentrated efforts of highly specialized teams.
8. Emergency	An acute and life-threatening problem that requires prompt and effective therapy and management for survival or to avoid permanent disability.
9. Chronic disability	A physical or functional disability of such long duration as to effectively remove the patient from the mainstream of society (e.g., physical handicaps, chronic diseases, degenerative diseases, aging).
10. Preventable ill	An illness that can be prevented by appropriate anticipatory steps such as immunization (e.g., smallpox) or public-health measures (e.g., water contamination).
11. Epidemic ill	A disease that characteristically spreads rapidly and affects large numbers of people unless effective action is taken.
12. Environmental ill	A dysfunction or disability resulting from environmental threats such as air pollution (bronchitis), water pollution (mercury poisoning), noise (hearing loss).
13. Occupational ill	A hazard to life and health resulting from an occupational environment (e.g., radiation, asbestos, solvents, accidents).
14. Psychosocial ill	An increased susceptibility to illness attributable in whole or in part to socioeconomic conditions.
15. Mental illness	A mental instability or debility of any sort (e.g., psychosis, neurosis, personality disturbance).

The term "sui-sickness" is intended to convey the self-destructive implications of many voluntary actions or urges. The "mal" in mini-mal is taken from the French word for sickness (as in mal de mer), and the "mini" indicates slight severity. Such functional disturbances are extremely common and extend well beyond the few examples listed in Table 2.3. Common ills and midi-mals are ailments of somewhat greater severity and significance. Mendi-mals are conditions for which available treatment is remedial or supportive but not curative. The remaining categories are self-explanatory from the definitions.

Distribution of Responsibility for Disabilities

The basic incentive for developing the terms and definitions of Table 2.3 was to provide a rational basis for the distribution of responsibility for different levels of illness. The fifteen categories of disease and disability are arranged in a circular array in Figure 2.5 to facilitate the achievement of a broad perspective in viewing their interactions.

Patient Sector

Conditions included under mini-mals and common ills represent the very common disturbances that interfere with the quality of life (usually temporarily) and rarely if ever pose significant threats to life or limb. They generally lack effective therapy capable of changing the progress or course of the ailment. As a rule patients with these conditions depend upon their own initiative or that of their immediate family to provide treatment (self-care). They sometimes seek the services of paramedical personnel. Patients suffering from most (if not all) of these illnesses derive little or no benefit from consulting physicians or entering the health-care system.

For example, the effectiveness of therapy obtained from pharmacists (over the counter) for colds and "flu" is clearly competitive with prescriptions from physicians. None are very effective. Glasses or hearing aids are not necessarily prescribed by physicians. Medical management of many annoying musculoskeletal disorders (arthritis, low back pain, etc.) is disappointing and ineffective, so that chiropractors and masseurs can still make a good living. Traditionally the health-care system is neither equipped nor geared to manage effectively mini-mals and common ills,

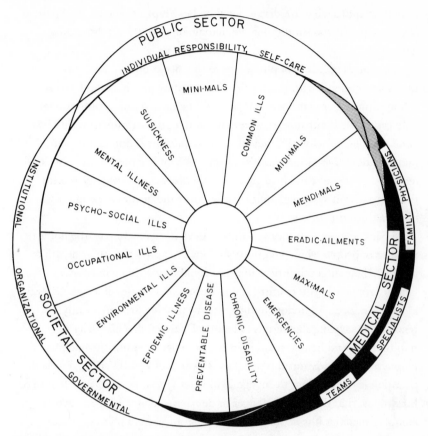

Figure 2.5 The fifteen different categories of health problems listed in Table 2.3 are arranged in a radiating pattern to indicate which can be considered the responsibility of the individual (public sector), of the medical sector, and of the organizations and agencies of society. Responsibility for the management of illness is shared at the junctures (as indicated by the overlapping regions at the circumference of the circle).

but other approaches are discouraged by health professionals. The patient often assumes responsibility for the management of these ailments by default.

The typical response of physicians to this situation is to focus on the fact that a few patients with these mild ailments may also have underlying serious illnesses or complications that will be missed unless professional help is sought. If our resources were unlimited, this argument would be a valid basis for providing sufficient medical personnel and facilities to manage all of these illnesses. When some 20% of our population is seriously deprived of effective medical care for vital illnesses, however, it is clear that our current system cannot hope to cover the hordes of people with mini-mals and common ills.

Sui-sickness is a category specifically devised to encompass the fantastic number of people whose voluntary actions pose threats to their health or increase their susceptibility to illness. Probably the single most serious health problem in this country is the overuse of all types of drugs. Obesity, alcoholism, drug addiction, and persistent smoking are universally recognized as being dangerous to health. Drunken driving, drug habituation, and heavy smoking in the presence of chronic bronchitis or emphysema are advanced types of sui-sickness. An established American tradition is the freedom to engage in any activity, no matter how foolish or hazardous, that does not endanger or deprive someone else. In current complex societies it is no longer possible for an individual to undertake foolish and unnecessary risks without inflicting the consequences on others, particularly in defraying the costs.

Injuries are common in individuals who engage in hazardous sports such as mountain climbing, skiing, scuba diving, or solo sailing in open water. Participants expose themselves to hazards and expect society to pay for their indulgences. Mountain climbers endanger rescue parties. Recently a man attempted to row a boat to Hawaii, and taxpayers paid $30,000 for the Coast Guard rescue. Serious consideration should be given to specifically excluding the treatment of such injuries from any private or national insurance program in order to provide an economic deterrent against such recklessness. It seems only fair that participants should be forced to make financial payment or penalties for illnesses resulting from these activities, just as automobile-insurance schedules penalize drinking drivers or accident-prone individuals. Tolerance toward these activities is now indirectly supporting instead of actively discouraging them. More effective nationwide health education is needed to combat sui-sickness by expanding activities such as the antismoking campaign to cover other types of self-indulgent threats to health and welfare.

Medical Sector

The health-care delivery system of this country quite naturally concentrates on the many types of illness for which effective therapy significantly improves the state of the patient's health. Midi-mals are illnesses that derive some benefit from remedies that are not sufficiently developed to cure or eliminate the cause. Symptomatic relief, supportive treatment, reassurance, and sympathy are important features of their management. The patients may have underlying illnesses or may develop complications of significance. The responsibility for midi-mals is shared by patients for self-management and by physicians for excluding complications. This category of illness is an ideal example of a proper role for the physician's assistant, nurse-practitioner, or multiphasic screening facility. The patient can oversee the details of the management, while the paramedical personnel can provide an interface with physicians to protect the patient against unforeseen problems. The physician's time can thus be conserved until his unique training is clearly called for.

In recent years medical progress has provided a rapidly widening spectrum of recognizable illnesses for which effective therapy can be applied. These increasing levels of effectiveness affect the categories of mendi-mals, eradic-ailments, maxi-mals, and emergencies. Eradic-ailments include conditions in which the source or cause of the ailment can be removed, repaired, or replaced by effective therapy (e.g., specific antibiotics, hormone replacement, reparative or reconstructive surgery). Maxi-mals involve intensive care, employing specialized teams and backed by sophisticated equipment, often providing dramatic life-saving services. Emergency services are designed to prolong the lives of individuals with acute life-threatening conditions that require prompt action, and commonly involve teams capable of rapid transportation and communication. Effective interaction and cooperation among societal service organizations (firemen, police, military helicopters, and communications networks) is required to provide effective emergency service in both urban and rural settings, and to this extent the responsibility for emergency services must be shared by the medical sector and the societal sector, as indicated schematically by the overlap in Figure 2.5.

Societal Sector

Many different kinds of illness have such scope or magnitude that they *must* be managed by organizations or governmental agencies rather than by patients themselves or members of the health team. Emergency services are a prime example. Chronic illnesses also produce patients, physically handicapped by crippling disease, accidents, or war, who must be cared for at home, in public institutions, or in veterans' hospitals depending upon the designation of responsibility. Inadequate attention has been directed to the costs and benefits that would result from an investment in the handicapped that would permit a larger proportion to be self-supporting instead of a drain on the public purse (see Chapter 7). The closing of many tuberculosis hospitals and sanataria is a prime example of the rewards of scientific progress in the management of debilitating diseases for which societal and medical sectors share responsibility. Another sign of success is the recent discontinuance of requirements for smallpox vaccination for many international travelers. However, the dangers of complacency are made clear by the rising incidence of the venereal diseases, diphtheria, and other illnesses for which management is so effective that complete elimination is theoretically possible. Treatable diseases that recur in epidemic proportions are a tragedy and a challenge that must stimulate effective action through the mobilization of whatever resources are necessary to reverse the trends. Experience has clearly demonstrated that an investment in the control of such diseases provides such great rewards that we cannot afford to fail in our efforts at suppression.

The increased hazards to health that result from deterioration of our environment pose problems of such diversity and extent that they can be attacked effectively only by governmental agencies (federal, state, and local). Respiratory diseases approaching epidemic proportions are a partial result of air pollution and a case in point. The accumulation of substances in air and water (e.g., mercury, sulphur, radioactive materials) can only be monitored and controlled by large and powerful agencies. Occupational environments account for an important subset of environmental problems, but must be countered by different measures and different institutions (e.g., labor unions) as well as by the policies, statutes, and agencies of government.

That there are important psychosocial components of illness is indicated by the high incidence of disease and disability among minorities and disadvantaged groups. The increased susceptibility to illness attributable to depressed socioeconomic status is a problem that cannot be effectively attacked by either the individuals involved or the health-care community. The prime responsibility for such problems must be accepted by the appropriate agencies of government, which must create and carry through effective programs to elevate the general human condition of these people. Efforts at providing them with improved health care will never be fully rewarding unless they are combined with programs to improve their financial, educational, and environmental condition.

Mental Illness

Mental illness includes a wide range of disturbances extending from overt psychoses, through psychoneuroses, to personality problems. This wide scope involves an overlap between societal responsibility and individual responsibility, as indicated in Figure 2.5. The diagnosis of mental illness is more subjective than exact, and the various forms of therapy utilized are by no means universally successful. For this reason the statistics regarding the incidence of mental illness are somewhat soft. Coming full circle in Figure 2.5, the proximity of mental illness and sui-sickness illustrates the importance of recognizing shared responsibility between society and the individual. Society must provide expanded and more effective health education in these areas and individuals must exhibit greater restraint in their own voluntary action to reduce the hazards to themselves and their fellow men.

Distribution of Illness and Concentration of Health-Care Resources

The wheel of health care in Figure 2.5 was designed to provide one basis for assessing the needs, requirements, and responsibilities for health care in a broad perspective. The compartments in the wheel are of equal size, but the incidences of the illnesses contained in them are grossly different. Exact data concerning the true incidences of ailments are not available, but ailments that are relatively mild (common ills) overwhelmingly predominate in the statistics. There must also be an extremely large number of individuals affected by mini-mals and sui-sickness, but again reliable numbers are elusive. Despite these deficiencies Figure 2.6A was prepared to illustrate the generally accepted impression that those ailments that fall primarily within the patient sector dominate the total incidence of current disease and disability.

At the moment the effectiveness of some of the most popular remedies for the common cold has been questioned by both medical authorities and the Food and Drug Administration. A somewhat larger investment by both government and private enterprise in more effective remedies for common ills appears fully warranted on any scale of cost and benefit. The pent-up demand for the care of common ailments could otherwise engulf the health-care system as national health insurance opens the floodgates.

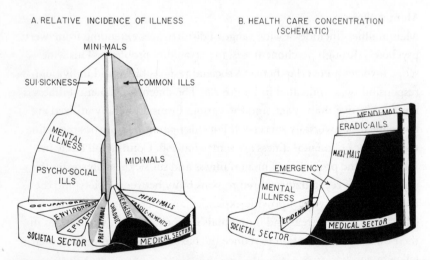

Figure 2.6 The highest incidence of health problems is found among the categories in the public sector of Figure 2.5, for which individual patients commonly assume primary responsibility (A). The major concentrations of health personnel and facilities in the medical sector are oriented primarily toward ailments known to be susceptible to remedial therapy (B). Subsequent chapters deal with proposed mechanisms for responding to this major discrepancy between A and B.

The current health-care system is oriented very heavily toward the categories extending from midi-mals through emergencies in Figure 2.5. These represent the categories for which personnel, facilities, research, and resources are predominantly allocated in the medical sector. To a significant degree they constitute conditions that have a lesser incidence but for which there is a greater prospect for positive improvement by proper care.

The presently constituted health-care system of this country is sorely stretched to meet current demands. Federally supported health insurance will present to enormous numbers of people who currently manage their own mild illnesses the opportunity to gain access to professional care that will appear artificially cheap or apparently free (see Chapter 3). European countries that have adopted national insurance or national health services have uniformly experienced such a deluge of patients overwhelming their health-care systems with illnesses previously managed by self-care. Steps should be taken promptly to protect our laboring health-care system from inundation with patients who will benefit little or not at all by their contact with health professionals.

Availability of Manpower in a Service-Oriented Society

Health-care delivery is primarily a service, and its key element is trained manpower. Serious shortages of natural resources are obvious on all sides, but the one ingredient that is in abundant surplus is manpower. Excess people is a worldwide problem, and its solution in the industrialized nations seems to be the evolution of a *service-oriented* society that will effectively utilize available human resources for the well-being and welfare of the population as a whole.

Surplus People

The developed nations of the world have proceeded in a sequence from agricultural to industrialized society mainly through mechanization. For example, the toil of more than 60% of the labor force was required to supply the United States with food until the latter part of the nineteenth century. Today mechanization and enlarged acreage allows about 6% of the labor force to produce food surpluses. (In contrast some under-

developed countries require as much as 80% of the working population merely for subsistence levels of food production.) An enormous
increase in productivity per worker has been the major result of the
agricultural revolution in this country. The freedom it gave to a large
fraction of our labor force permitted the transition to an industrial society
which has provided the average American citizen with a degree of
affluence that would have been the envy of royal families of earlier times.
As mechanization of goods and products proceeded, the steadily increasing
output per worker allowed an ever-greater utilization of personnel in
service types of enterprises. The further expansion of industrial production
is sharply limited by growing shortages of raw materials and energy,
coupled with threats to the environment stemming from pollution and
solid-waste production. These are compelling reasons to funnel an even
greater proportion of available "people-power" into service-oriented
activities that are specifically designed to improve the quality of life for all
citizens with minimal contamination of our fragile environment.

The Growth of Service Functions
The trend toward expansion of service-oriented activities has become well
established over the past twenty years. Service-producing activities include
personal services such as health care, transportation, public utilities,
wholesale and retail trade, finance, insurance, real estate, and government. Goods-production, involving mining, agriculture, contract
construction, and manufacturing, employed about the same number of
workers as the service functions in 1950. In the ensuing twenty years
employment in service functions has expanded by more than 20 million
people. Projections to 1980 suggest that services will then employ 65% of
the labor force, almost twice the number of people producing goods. These
trends are significant because health care is preeminent among the services
in terms of demand, expenditures, and unmet needs.

The growing demands for research and development, education, and
health services, as well as for the processing of all kinds of paper work in
these enterprises, will produce a rapidly increasing number of white-collar
jobs, while the number of blue-collar and farm jobs will grow slowly if at
all. Professional and technical workers (more than 11.1 million), including
highly trained personnel such as teachers, engineers, health personnel,

accountants, and others, will constitute the fastest growing occupational group (with an increase of possibly 40%) during the next ten years.

Summary

The accelerating rates of change of modern societies demand longer-range planning and assessment of the consequences of various courses of action. Futures research is providing a variety of new techniques to produce more consistent and reliable projections of future developments, particularly on technological matters. But these processes do not necessarily lead to sound choices or optimal pathways to avoid immediate obstacles in progressing into the future. An alternative approach is the concept of *creating desirable futures* by defining optimal long-range goals for a future ten to twenty years hence, identifying the many options for reaching these goals, and evaluating their advantages, disadvantages, and consequences. It is intended that the combination of clearly defined goals and well-evaluated options will be utilized in appropriate decisions at many different decision points during the ensuing years.

Predictable changes in society will probably influence the kinds of options that can be selected. For example, the most advanced nations are in a transition from an industrial, product-oriented phase into a service-oriented phase in which a great majority of the labor force will be engaged in rendering service rather than producing tangible goods. This projection indicates that health, education, and communication will be among the most important activities into which the labor force will be funneled during the next decades. Enormous amounts of human energy can be effectively utilized to improve the quality of life for thousands of young, old, disadvantaged, and handicapped people who need, but cannot acquire, necessary services.

The whole health-care delivery system needs to be considered by systems analysis and long-range planning. Definitions of health and sickness need categorization indicating both the levels of severity, the principal sites of care, and the distribution of responsibility for management among the parties involved (the public, the medical sector, and the societal sector).

References

1. Anne R. Somers. 1971. *Health Care in Transition: Directions for the Future.* Chicago: Hospital Research and Educational Trust.
2. Rashi Fein. 1967. *The Doctor Shortage: An Economic Diagnosis.* Studies in Social Economics. Washington, D.C.: The Brookings Institution.
3. Richard M. Magraw. 1966. *Ferment in Medicine: A Study of the Essence of Medical Practice and of Its New Dilemmas.* Philadelphia: Saunders.
4. Edward J. Burger. 1974. Health and health services in the United States: A perspective and a discussion of some issues. *Ann. Intern. Med.* 80:645–650.
5. *Report of the National Advisory Commission on Health Manpower.* 1967. Vol. 1. Washington, D.C.: U.S. Government Printing Office.
6. Abraham B. Bergman, S.W. Dassel, and Ralph J. Wedgewood. 1966. Time-motion studies of practicing pediatricians. *Pediatrics* 38:254–263.
7. Henry K. Silver, L.D. Ford, and S.G. Stearly. 1967. A program to increase health care for children: The pediatric nurse practitioner program. *Pediatrics* 39:756–760.
8. The New York City Planning Commission. 1969. *Plan for New York City.* Vol. 1. *Critical Issues.* Cambridge, Mass.: The MIT Press.
9. S.E. Harris. 1964. *The Economics of American Medicine.* New York: Macmillan.
10. H.E. Klarman. 1965. *The Economics of Health.* New York: Columbia University Press.
11. Homer J. Hagedorn and James J. Dunlop. 1965. Health care delivery as a social system: Inhibitions and constraints on change. *Proc. IEEE* 57:1894–1900.

3
Concepts of Cost/Benefit and Value-Added Applied to Health Care

The costs of health services have reached such high levels that they are beyond the reach of a large segment of the population, particularly those not covered by insurance or other third-party payments. As the upward spiral of health-care costs continues, there is growing need for the assignment of priorities to insure that resources are allocated in a manner that is in the best interests of both patients and society as a whole.

Priorities require criteria and definitions of health care that are clear and specific (see Figure 2.5). On theoretical grounds one appropriate basis for judgment would be an estimate of cost-effectiveness. Unfortunately the growing need for a more effective evaluation of cost/benefit relationships occurs at a time when neither the costs nor the results of health services can be precisely evaluated.

Cost/Benefit Relations

In a society dominated by a free market the balance between costs and benefits is normally achieved through the process of supply and demand. Expenditures for drugs, personnel, facilities, and materials can, in fact, be assessed by standard accounting procedures (Figure 3.1). However, the nonprofit status of most of the voluntary hospitals has not stimulated tight cost-accounting procedures. There is a common tendency for the charges on common laboratory procedures and unit costs to be elevated, so that patients with mild or moderate diseases help to pay for the costs of the more sophisticated elements of health-care delivery. Despite these uncontrollable factors estimates can be developed of the funds expended for the management of various kinds of disease either in hospitals or outside.

The problem of quantitatively assessing the *benefits* derived from the ministrations of health professionals is even more troublesome.[1] The monetary equivalents of life expectancy and health have always been regarded as beyond estimate, and economic value cannot be assigned to the worth of "reassurance," the "relief of symptoms," or the need for "prognosis" (Figure 3.1). So long as the health-care delivery system

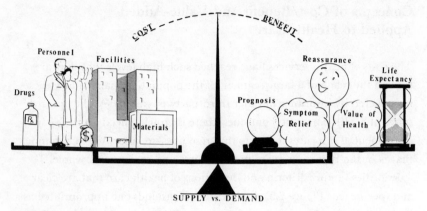

SUPPLY vs. DEMAND

Figure 3.1 An economic balance between cost and benefit of a service is established by supply and demand in a free and unregulated economy. The cost of health care can be estimated from the utilization of resources such as drugs, personnel, facilities, and other materials. The benefits realized by patients in terms of life expectancy, restoration of health, relief of symptoms, prognosis, or reassurance are highly personal and lacking in economic equivalent. The need to develop more meaningful priorities requires improved evaluation of the relative benefits derived from various alternatives as a basis for determining the most effective and equitable distribution of limited resources. From R. F. Rushmer, *Medical Engineering; Projections for Health Care Delivery* (New York: Academic Press, 1970), with permission of the publisher.

operates on the basic assumption that its benefits are impossible to define, the possibility of developing priorities with solid meaning is open to serious question. Indeed there was no need to assign numerical values to "benefits" so long as expenditures on health were relatively small and the laws of supply and demand were functioning without distortion. Now, however, the large-scale involvement of third-party payments obscures the cost and upsets the natural constraints on utilization that result from direct payment for services. It is no longer possible to assume that the amount of money a consumer pays for a service establishes its free-market value.

Artificially Cheap—Apparently Free

The sharing of costs for health care by means of either insurance or federal subsidy is a valuable mechanism for equalizing wealth and opportunity among the citizenry. It provides essential services under conditions that make them apparently free or artificially cheap. Subsidies tend to create an expanded demand for services that cannot be fully met. The inevitable consequence is congestion of the service and waiting lines. If the quantity of health services cannot be increased sufficiently to meet the demand, society must then face agonizing decisions about criteria for priorities to determine which patients should benefit from the health-care system. This suggests that access to health care will always be denied some segments of society.

There is a need to face up to the challenge of expanding those aspects of health-care delivery that can be demonstrated to be most effective. Research resources must be funneled toward improved therapeutic capabilities for those conditions that are common but currently lack effective therapeutic measures. The overall problem is compounded by our long tradition of expecting the physician to do something for each patient, which tends to obscure the fact that effective therapeutic procedures are not available for a very large number of common illnesses.

Cost/Benefit Categories

Cost/benefit balances can be evaluated subjectively in the manner indicated for some sample categories in Figure 3.2. For example, third-party payment mechanisms obscure the actual cost to the patient and therefore leave the impression that any degree of benefit is worthwhile (upper left). If a patient pays only a modest sum for several days spent in a hospital in comfortable surroundings for a minor illness, he regards the benefit as quite adequate. So long as insurance or federal funds are available, there is little or no urgency felt by anyone to evaluate critically the relationship between the cost and the effectiveness of the services rendered.

A realistic benefit can be clearly visualized in those cases where a disease can be prevented by a simple and cheap procedure such as vaccination (Figure 3.2, lower left). Similarly there can be no question about the benefit derived when therapy has been developed to a point where the cause of a major disease can be eliminated or suppressed. When a patient recovers more rapidly from a disease or disability through the direct actions of the health-care professionals, the benefit is clearly recognizable by all concerned. On this basis a favorable cost/benefit ratio is obvious to the patient who is aided by the effective action of a health-care team.

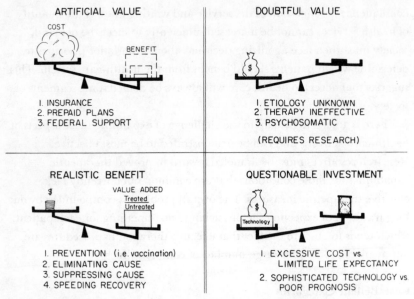

ARTIFICIAL VALUE
1. INSURANCE
2. PREPAID PLANS
3. FEDERAL SUPPORT

DOUBTFUL VALUE
1. ETIOLOGY UNKNOWN
2. THERAPY INEFFECTIVE
3. PSYCHOSOMATIC
(REQUIRES RESEARCH)

REALISTIC BENEFIT
1. PREVENTION (i.e. vaccination)
2. ELIMINATING CAUSE
3. SUPPRESSING CAUSE
4. SPEEDING RECOVERY

QUESTIONABLE INVESTMENT
1. EXCESSIVE COST vs. LIMITED LIFE EXPECTANCY
2. SOPHISTICATED TECHNOLOGY vs. POOR PROGNOSIS

Figure 3.2 Cost/benefit relationships can be indicated for certain circumstances. For example, third-party payments make health care seem artificially cheap or apparently free, obscuring the real costs and making any benefit seem worthwhile to the patient. Prevention, cure, and speeded recovery as a direct result of therapy is a clear-cut benefit of high order. The cost/benefit ratio is doubtful in treating illnesses for which the etiology is unknown or therapy is ineffective. These require additional research. Sophisticated and expensive treatment of illnesses that have poor prognosis suggests that the investment may be debatable when other, more attractive options must be neglected.

When the cause of a disease is unknown, or therapy is ineffective, or the problem is psychosomatic in origin, the value of the services provided by the health-care system is incalculable. There is certainly a clear need for research into the large number of conditions for which health care provides benefits of doubtful value. But how are we to assign a value to tests and therapeutic programs that have doubtful effects?

The cost/benefit ratio may also be unclear for a large and growing category of serious or life-threatening diseases that are managed through the use of highly sophisticated techniques and technologies (intensive-care units, artificial dialysis for kidney failure, radical surgery). There is no precedent for assessing the relative importance of such investments in critical comparison with alternative uses for the same amounts of money.

We may be forced to develop criteria for gauging the benefit on some reasonable basis and to allocate our resources to do the greatest good for the greatest number. Efforts should be directed toward logical criteria for comparing potential rewards from investments in various areas of research and health care. Two different but related mechanisms will now be tentatively proposed for consideration, primarily to illustrate that the concepts of cost/benefit ratios and value-added can indeed be applied to some extent in this area.

Some Criteria for Evaluating Cost-Effectiveness or Cost/Benefit

One possible method of evaluating the effectiveness of medical care might be based on the relationship between the specificity of the diagnosis and the nature of the therapeutic results.[2] In Figure 3.3 diagnostic specificity ranges from "no diagnosis" to quantitative tests that provide consistent and specific diagnostic reliability. The range of therapeutic results is indicated along the left margin of Figure 3.3 and extends from mere reassurance by the physician through symptomatic relief and the reduction of complications, to the elimination of the cause and the prevention of illness. There is little basis for doubting that a patient will receive major benefit from the health-care delivery system if the cause of his illness is either suppressed, eliminated, or prevented. Effective criteria for evaluating the success of the treatment must, however, be based on a high degree of diagnostic specificity. For example, the evaluation of success in the treatment of mental illness, fever of unknown origin, or athero-sclerosis is very unreliable because of a lack of diagnostic specificity. Claims for therapeutic effectiveness for conditions whose cause is unknown may be defined as "quackery."

On the basis of Figure 3.3 the relationship between a high level of medical diagnostic specificity and effective therapy can be designated as a *major benefit,* while an *intermediate benefit* would be indicated where reliable diagnosis is accompanied by some definite improvement derived from the therapy. A *minor benefit* would result when the physician is able to provide only reassurance, prognosis, and some symptomatic relief.

The concepts presented in Figure 3.3 are intended to indicate that at least a start could and should be made in providing this kind of assessment. The remainder of this chapter will be devoted to a consideration of the

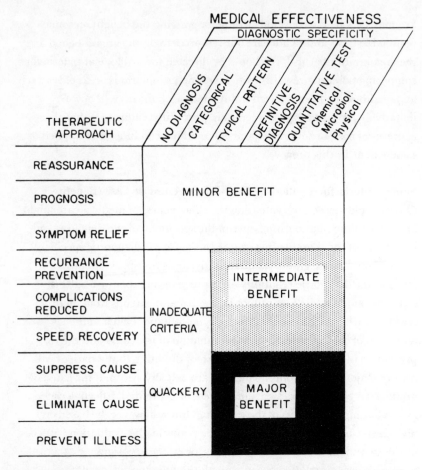

Figure 3.3 A mechanism for evaluating relative "benefit" is proposed for consideration. The highest "benefit" from health services is for ailments that can be positively (even quantitatively) diagnosed and that can also be prevented, eliminated, or actively suppressed by treatment (black area). Intermediate benefit is attained for diagnosed illnesses by actively speeding recovery, reducing complications, or preventing recurrences (stippled area). Minor benefit is available through symptomatic relief and the process of reassurance and prognosis, despite diagnostic specificity (white area). The effectiveness of therapy cannot be gauged in the absence of a definitive diagnosis.

benefit side of the cost/benefit relationship, necessarily based on subjective impressions more than on objective scales or quantitative measures. It must be obvious by now that a most important factor in the evaluation must be the effectiveness of available therapy.

Relative effectiveness of therapies for various categories of illness
The extent to which the actions of health professionals favorably affect the course of a disease or disability is often difficult to evaluate, particularly among the many abnormal states lacking quantitative diagnostic tests. Subjective evaluation of patient response to a treatment is rendered suspect or unreliable by the "placebo" effect of the ministrations of health professionals, even when they are recognized as incapable of alleviating pathophysiological processes. Assessment of treatment is even more unreliable in patients with ailments of uncertain etiology, subjective diagnostic signs, and nonspecific methods of management.

Definitive therapy. An ever-growing number of diseases respond to definitive therapy by either preventive methods or curative treatments that suppress or eliminate the basic causes of disability (Figure 3.4). Nutritional diseases have largely disappeared in this country due to the general improvement in the standard of living and the availability of essential foodstuffs during the past several decades. Conditions such as scurvy, beriberi, pellagra, rickets, goiter, and other dietary-deficiency states are extremely uncommon except among the poorest segments of the population. Additional examples are communicable diseases such as cholera, plague, malaria, smallpox, diphtheria, typhoid-paratyphoid fevers, poliomyelitis, and the venereal diseases. In general these controllable conditions have succumbed to large-scale socioeconomic developments or massive public-health programs. Similarly the environmental threats of air and water pollution and work hazards such as exposure to radiation or noxious chemicals constitute conditions that require efforts at prevention through effective action by the societal sector.

Curable diseases. Curable diseases are exemplified by the myriad forms of infection that have proved susceptible to antibiotics, including streptococcal infections, pneumonia, meningitis, dysenteries, and tuberculosis. There are by now well-established surgical techniques for the excision of tumors, local infections, and obstructions, and for the repair or

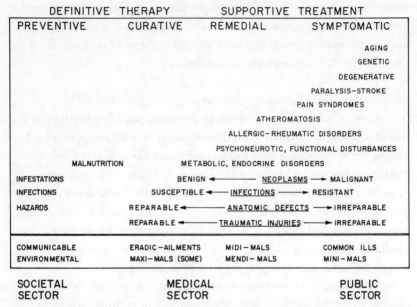

Figure 3.4 The relative effectiveness of therapy is indicated for selected categories of ailments. Definitive therapy is exemplified by those conditions that can be either effectively prevented by the societal sector or cured by direct action of the medical sector. Ailments subject only to supportive therapy and symptomatic relief greatly outnumber those that succumb to definitive therapy.

reconstruction of congenital malformations of the heart, gastrointestinal tract, or genitourinary tract. The continuing development of new tissue and organ substitutes presages future replacements of increasing complexity. All of these conditions can justifiably be listed under preventive or curative categories in Figure 3.4.

Supportive treatment. The total number of preventable or curable diseases and disturbances is substantial but still represents a relatively small proportion of the health hazards that affect mankind. Indeed rapid scientific progress may well be eliciting new diseases or subcategories faster than old ones are succumbing. For example, environmental hazards and the causes of trauma have been greatly expanded by modern technologies. Speeding vehicles contribute to both environmental deterioration and the added incidence of violent accidents. Dramatic successes in the control of many infectious diseases still leave large numbers of viruses, bacteria, and protozoa that are resistive or unresponsive to antibiotics. Similarly, benign tumors are subject to curative therapy, but more malignant cancers must be managed by remedial or supportive means with much less prospect of certain cure.

Remedial management. Many familiar ailments are favorably influenced by remedial measures even when the cause is unknown. Common examples include hypertension, peptic ulcers, psychoneurotic and functional disturbances, allergic and rheumatic disorders, atheromatosis, and the distressing-pain syndromes. Certain metabolic disorders can be effectively handled by endocrine-replacement therapy, as in the case of diabetes, hypothyroidism, and other hormonal imbalances. These approaches can hardly be regarded as curative since the original source of the problem is not under attack.

Many patients with mild, moderate, and severe ailments can receive only symptomatic management, which includes efforts to alleviate distress and provide support and sympathy. Obvious examples include the disabilities associated with aging, genetic diseases, degenerative conditions, paralysis, pain syndromes, osteoarthritis, and many common ills or mini-mals of the sort described in Chapter 2.

Illness with Highest Incidence

The National Center for Health Statistics of the U.S. Public Health Service collects enormous quantities of information regarding the health status of many segments of the American population. During the year following July 1, 1967, data was collected from 42,000 households containing about 134,000 persons by weekly interviews conducted by trained personnel of the U.S. Bureau of Census. During that year the incidence of acute illness or injuries (involving medical attention or reduced daily activity) was 368,356,000 (a rate of 189.4 conditions for each hundred persons per year). Common colds were responsible for over half of the acute conditions (56% of the total). During the twelve-month period an estimated 80 million conditions were reported as influenza-like illness, an incidence rate of 41.3 conditions per 100 persons per year. These samples were elicited from standard metropolitan statistical areas (SMSA). The data from these areas have been found to be representative of those in metropolitan areas and in nonfarm areas outside of the study areas.

The combined incidence of cholera, plague, malaria, diphtheria, smallpox, poliomyelitis, rheumatic fever, typhoid, and parasites is presented on the left side of Figure 3.5 and shows the extent to which "previous problems," including major plagues and epidemics, have been controlled.

Samples of major medical problems are presented in the next highest column, respiratory infections and trauma representing the largest segments. These respiratory infections refer to specific bacterial infestations, most of which are susceptible to treatment with antibiotics. In addition the incidence of venereal disease, cystitis, pregnancy complications, functional bowel disease, myocardial infarction, hypertension, allergies, paralysis and stroke, peptic ulcers, bowel hemmorrhage, and

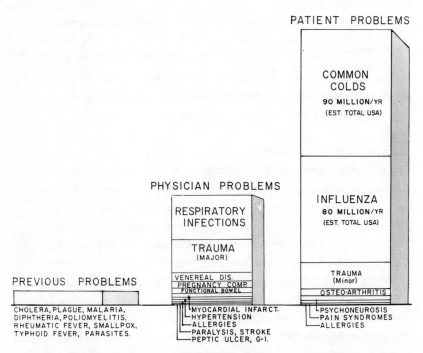

Figure 3.5 Preventable diseases characteristically become rare, often almost to the vanishing point. Notable exceptions are the venereal diseases, which are currently increasing in incidence for other reasons. The diseases included as physician problems are dominated by respiratory infections and trauma, and the familiar diseases appear relatively rare in comparison. The very high incidence of common ailments designated as patient problems include major components of common colds, influenza, and minor trauma, with lesser numbers of distressing and debilitating disabilities. Compiled from data from National Center for Health Statistics.[6]

venous disease totaled some 77 million cases for the year of the sampling.

The very high incidence of common colds and "influenza-like" illnesses is indicated in the tallest column; their combined incidence of approximately 170 million cases per year is more than 20 times the number of patients included under previous problems. Minor trauma, osteoarthritis, psychoneuroses, back pain, and allergies are conditions that appear in lesser frequency, but are major causes of disability and suffering. The common complaint that modern medical science has made great strides in the management of epidemic diseases and in the development of sophisticated diagnostic and therapeutic equipment and yet has done very little for the cure or prevention of the common cold is emphasized by this illustration.

The Concept of Value Added by Health Care

One way to measure the success of a process is to estimate or compute the increase in value that results from its application. This is the method employed in economics to assess the effectiveness of industrialization; it is generally applied to processes for the production of goods that have monetary value. For example, raw materials gain enhanced value as they are processed and converted into products of increasing worth.

This approach is not ordinarily applied to a service for which the economic value is difficult to specify. In health care the patient is the raw material, and the process is health-care delivery. If we wish to become more objective and quantitative about the contribution of health-care delivery, the benefit derived by the patient must be estimated by a comparison with the results expected in an "average untreated case." For example, if either the duration of the illness or the resultant degree of disability can be specified for some sample of patients who do not have access to modern medicine, the effectiveness of therapy by health professionals may then be assessed by direct comparison. Unfortunately the characteristics of the course of untreated illnesses have rarely been documented for many reasons, including wide variability among different individuals suffering from the same illness. Furthermore patients without access to health care undoubtedly have other major socioeconomic problems that would complicate evaluation. These uncertainties preclude quantitative comparisons but do not prevent a search for gross differences.

The criteria for the value added by medical management can be helpfully expressed in terms of the reduction in duration or recurrence of the disease in treated patients as compared with informed guesses about untreated patients (Figure 3.6). An estimate as to the *degree* of disability in the treated patient as compared to a standard untreated patient might represent a second approach to evaluation. A third approach might be a quantitative estimate of the reduction in the residual consequences of illness. Fourth, for epidemiological purposes an increase in life expectancy for groups of treated patients as opposed to untreated samples might be useful. Finally, in recent years the economic significance of treatment has been estimated by translating the time lost by individuals as a result of disease to dollar amounts.

This process could be extended to a general comparison of the economic significance of the treatment of illness if it were possible to establish a reliable data base regarding the courses of the many illnesses that lack effective treatment. Examples of this process are extremely rare. Harry Weintrob and Elliot Ratnor[3] have reported a cost/benefit analysis for two respiratory intensive-care units and have extrapolated their results to the total population based on the 33,000 deaths per year from chronic obstructive lung disease. They collected data indicating that the mortality rates for such patients prior to intensive care units was 55%, which was interpreted to mean that some 60,000 people had severe, chronic respiratory disease. On the basis of such assumptions they estimated that 22,800 lives could be prolonged by respiratory intensive care at a cost of $21,000 each, with an estimated addition of 148,000 life-years. Although both the assumptions and conclusions in this particular study may be questioned, it constitutes one of the few comparisons of treated to untreated patients as an indication of the value added by health services.

Contributions of Various Therapeutic Approaches

The Value Added by Prevention
Preventable disease tends to disappear. The devastating epidemic diseases of the past have become so rare that many physicians can go through years

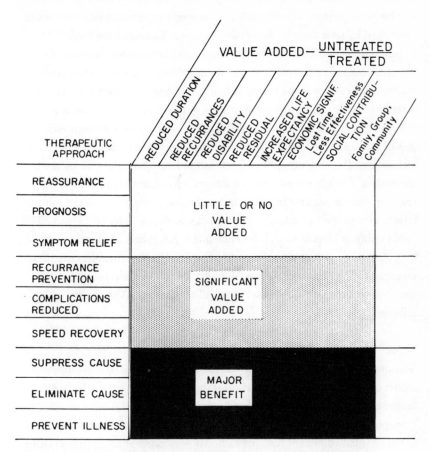

Figure 3.6 The concept of value-added could theoretically be applied to therapy by comparing treated patients with the expected course of illness without treatment, with respect to duration, recurrences, disability, life expectancy, economic significance, and potential social contribution of the patient. The vertical scale presents the levels of therapeutic effectiveness in the left-hand column of Figure 3.3.

of practice without ever seeing a single case. Despite our inability to arrive at a basis for judging priorities there is one concept that appears to be fully supported by past history. According to Lewis Thomas,[4] the high technology of medicine that results from a genuine understanding of disease mechanisms is relatively inexpensive and relatively easy to deliver. "Offhand, I cannot think of any important human disease that medicine possesses the capacity to prevent or cure outright in which the cost of the technology is itself the major problem. The price is never as high as the cost of managing the same disease was during the early stages of ineffective technology. If a case of typhoid fever had to be managed today by the best methods of 1935, it would run to a staggering expense." Similarly no one really questions the cost in effort and technology that has resulted in the virtual elimination of many of the nutritional deficiencies of the past. The "white plague" has been so fully controlled that tuberculosis sanataria and hospitals have closed all over the nation. Such accomplishments present an exceedingly important lesson, namely that prevention requires development of sufficient knowledge and technology to stamp out or cure ailments.

Value Added by Definitive Therapy
The progress of medical science that has allowed physicians to eliminate causes or to speed recovery constitutes the second-highest level of value added by the health-care system. Destructive surgery has been an effective example in this category for many years. The ability to remove tumors and to excise infected organs (in appendicitis) or abnormal concretions (kidney stones) has been around for many years. More recently the techniques of surgery have been extended to the repair and reconstruction of tissues and organs, ranging from the repair of hernias (an age-old technique) to the delicate restoration of the internal structures in children with severe congenital anomalies. Reconstructive surgery now also involves the replacement of normal structures and functions by artificial substitutes. Substitution therapy is also an effective mechanism for the management of hormonal deficiencies (diabetes and hypothyroidism), as is the utilization of specific biochemical substitutes for normally occurring substances. The techniques for management of life-threatening conditions have been greatly improved through the development of sophisticated intensive-care

units. A notable example is the remarkable reduction in fatalities resulting from war injuries on the battlefield.

Value Added by Supportive Therapy

Many of the major medical problems, such as those illustrated in Figure 3.4, can be neither prevented nor cured by the action of health professionals. One of the major roles of the physician is thus the management of complications and the attempt to sustain life during acute episodes and to reduce recurrences. An even clearer example is hypertension, in which the elevated blood pressure can be lowered by the continued administration of effective drugs and the incidence of complications such as heart failure or occlusion of the arteries to the brain can thereby be reduced. The paralysis that develops after a stroke is not greatly influenced by the actions of physicians with currently available techniques, and the rehabilitation of such patients presents problems of great complexity for which adequate solutions have not yet been developed. In contrast the medical and surgical treatment of peptic ulcers can effectively alter the course of the illness and facilitate the recovery of patients in easily demonstrated ways.

Value Added by Diagnosis without Effective Therapy

When a physician is confronted by a patient with a set of signs and symptoms, both parties regard the first step to be the establishment of a definitive diagnosis. This is regarded as an essential ingredient in the doctor-patient relationship, whether or not medical science has any effective therapy to offer. If the diagnosis is not rendered fairly obvious by the pattern of signs and symptoms, a relatively large expenditure of effort, time, and resources will often be devoted to its determination. This has become particularly evident with the automation of clinical laboratories, which provide extremely large quantities of information with little effort on the part of the patient and even less on the part of the physician. In the minds of many diagnostic testing is currently being overused, particularly in those instances where extensive routines are repeatedly employed with little prospect of effective therapy. The standard laboratory tests, automatically ordered whenever a patient enters a hospital, are now being supplemented by a wide variety of tests, many of which are unrewarding if insufficient discrimination is used in their selection. According to J.H.U. Brown and James Dickson,[5] clinical laboratories had batteries of tests limited to only about 12 biochemical determinations ten years ago. Today similar laboratories are being called upon to perform any one of 50 to 350 different types of analysis. About 500 million of these tests are now performed annually, and it is likely that this number will double over the next five years as it has every five years since 1946. The overuse of various forms of clinical testing has become so commonplace and so unrestrained that it contributes significantly to the soaring costs of medicine, but no one knows how much it really contributes to the health status of patients.

The annual checkup

For many years the medical profession has encouraged the general public to have "checkups" on an annual basis so that diseases can be detected at an early stage in their development, when they can be treated more economically and more effectively. According to Morgan, "the annual physical owes its popularity to the belief that certain diseases can be detected at a presymptomatic stage. As a consequence, appropriate—and, it is hoped, curative—therapy will be given earlier than usual. It is further implied that early diagnosis and treatment inevitably enhance the chance of cure. With one or two exceptions, the evidence to support this view is tenuous in the extreme" (*Hospital Tribune*, May 31, 1971). He warned against physicians being so busy examining asymptomatic patients who need no treatment that the patient who is genuinely ill with severe symptoms can obtain medical help only in a hospital emergency room. This dispute can be resolved only by much more specific information regarding the cost-effectiveness, cost/benefit, and value added as a result of the checkup procedures employed.

I suspect that a critical evaluation of unselected groups of routine annual checkups would prove them to be relatively unrewarding in relation to realistic costs. Indeed many aspects of the routine physical examination are no longer truly relevant to the incidence of disease as it exists today. For example, in the examination of the chest the physician routinely listens over the heart for the heart sounds and murmurs. The most significant finding from this process is a murmur that is related to defective heart valves. The traditional causes of defective heart valves are syphilis, rheumatic fever, and congenital heart disease. Syphilis and rheumatic fever have been so thoroughly controlled in recent years that the incidence of deformed valves from this source has become extremely small. In any of the three cases the deformity of the valve neither develops rapidly nor disappears, so that repeated examinations add nothing to the original finding. Similarly the physician consistently percusses the chest and listens to breath sounds. This process was originally intended to detect either pneumonia or tuberculosis. These ailments are now so extremely rare that the potential contribution of this step is relatively limited. A single chest x-ray taken at relatively infrequent intervals will do a far superior job of detecting the size of the heart and the status of the lungs. Neither percussion nor auscultation provides unique clues regarding the existence of more important problems such as atherosclerosis of the coronary arteries or common pulmonary disease.

The cost-effectiveness of the physical examination is difficult to evaluate, particularly since there is a very clear contribution to the welfare of the patient that stems from the reassurance, the personal contact, and the feeling of involvement between the patient and his physician. On the other hand a realistic assessment of the contribution of the physical examination to diagnostic accuracy can and should be attempted. Most annual checkups and virtually all admissions to hospitals are associated with a fairly routine set of laboratory determinations. Such physical examinations and laboratory determinations are required by an extremely wide variety of institutions, including life-insurance companies, employers, schools, and camps, in the course of a lifetime. These rituals contribute little or nothing to the welfare of the public.

The concept of multiphasic screening
The early detection of disease processes so that effective treatment can be instituted before functional or physical damage becomes manifest is a most attractive idea. It clearly stems from the "preventive maintenance" that is widely employed in preserving mechanical devices, including the family car. Indeed this concept has attracted so much attention and interest that it is commonly regarded as the next important trend in medicine. As a result techniques for rapidly and cheaply testing patients without signs or symptoms have been developed in an effort to discover and arrest incipient

problems. Included among these efforts are the development of Automated Multiphasic Health Testing Facilities with diagnostic procedures highly organized so that large amounts of data can be collected by devices in the hands of technicians.[7] The ambulatory client first undergoes a battery of tests and procedures conducted by paramedical personnel in an auto-mated multitest laboratory, and subsequently a physician reviews the multitest data, conducts a physical examination, and then proceeds in a traditional manner to diagnose, treat, and arrange follow-up procedures if called for.

Extensive experience has indicated that multiphasic testing can be an effective method of health surveillance, case detection of certain types of disease, and disease monitoring. Several inherent difficulties have also become evident. The tests that have been successfully automated and included in the series are not necessarily those that would be most specific and useful in the early detection of *treatable* diseases. For this reason substantial numbers of otherwise healthy people show evidence of ailments or disabilities for which therapy is not effective. The value added by the early recognition of conditions for which management is ineffectual is open to question.

In addition the standards for normality among such tests are fairly wide. Variations in test results for technical reasons often provide values that are "not within normal limits" but do not necessarily justify any definite diagnosis. This rather common problem cannot be ignored and calls for additional testing, often involving fruitless expense and unnecessary worry by the patient. The greatest single deterrent to the dominance of preventive maintenance in medicine is the fact that a large proportion of the illnesses that can be accurately diagnosed cannot be directly alleviated by the action of health professionals.

Cost-effectiveness estimates have been favorable when applied to large groups of individuals undergoing regular screening. Improved life expectancy and added productive years of impressive dimensions have been reported. For example, Morris Collen,[8] studying computer-aided multiphasic testing, found that four or five times as many test results could be obtained for the same cost as traditional methods. He cited data in which as many as 25% of all patients tested showed a significant abnormality on chest x-ray and/or electrocardiogram; 7.5%, hypertension;

5% of women, anemia; 3.3% of all patients, diabetes; one in 500 women over 50, breast cancer; and one in 5,000, parathyroid tumor. Some of these conditions respond well to therapy; others are more difficult to manage. In seven years of health surveillance in a controlled study, middle-aged males had a statistically significant reduction in disability and mortality, and a greater total earnings. Despite these favorable findings I would predict that a more critical evaluation of the value added by multiphasic screening would be disappointing.

There is basis for belief that the yield of automated multiphasic screening could be significantly improved by using various prescreening techniques or risk factors to concentrate into smaller populations persons with a greater likelihood of having the kinds of illness the tests are capable of disclosing (see Chapters 6 and 7). Selected elements of multiphasic-screening batteries could also be employed for health appraisal to help monitor the course of illnesses during chronic management.

The Value Added by "Doing Something"

A patient clearly derives benefits that are intangible but recognizable whenever a physician engages in some process intended to be for his benefit, even if the effect on the course of his illness is limited or absent. There is no question but that the "laying on of hands" has a distinctive and unique therapeutic significance, even in the course of a physical examination. Laboratory testing, either routine or specialized, also tends to provide both reassurance and the prospect of a prognosis and possibly successful therapeutic efforts. A prescription for a drug or a therapeutic procedure is almost the inevitable result of any visit to a physician with a presenting sign or symptom. A beneficial effect is generally recognized by a patient who takes a pill or follows a doctor's orders, even when the prescription or procedure is without therapeutic benefit. This well-recognized "placebo effect" is widely employed by physicians, to the obvious benefit of their patients, but it complicates even the most conscientious effort to assess the effectiveness of theoretically beneficial treatments. In our efforts to become more exact and scientific in our evaluation of medical success we might deprive patients of the undeniable but unmeasurable benefits gained by contact with health professionals, ingestion of impotent drugs, and application of palliative procedures. At least we must be candid and realistic in such judgments so that we do not engage in self-delusion. Caution must also be exercised to avoid the production of symptoms and signs in susceptible people as a direct result of well-intentioned therapeutic efforts.

Summary

This chapter has been designed to suggest possible criteria for consideration in establishing priorities for future planning. Analysis indicates that cost/benefit ratios and the determination of value-added are most favorable when illnesses can be prevented, cured, or alleviated by effective medical or surgical attack on a known cause (see Figure 3.3). The management or prevention of complications present a somewhat lower level of benefit. The diagnosis of ailments that cannot be effectively treated can help provide prognosis or reassurance but cannot influence the course of the underlying illness.

The health professions have not yet been challenged to examine their diagnostic and therapeutic efforts critically in such a cold light. Realistic incentives have been lacking to consider methods of economizing on either the costs to individual patients or the total costs of care to the general public. Priorities are now needed, however, and the next chapter will be devoted to a consideration of some of our current priorities and also some of the unmet needs that are receiving grossly inadequate attention and support.

References

1. Robert F. Rushmer. 1972. *Medical Engineering: Projections for Health Care Delivery.* New York: Academic.
2. Robert F. Rushmer. 1971. The filter and the gatekeeper functions. In *Proceedings. Conference on a Critical Analysis of the Cost-Effectiveness of Multiphasic Screening*, eds., Stephen R. Yarnall and Jay S. Wakefield. Seattle: Medical Computer Services Association.
3. Harry Weintrob and Elliot Z. Ratnor. 1972. Cost benefit analysis of the respiratory intensive care unit (RICU) for respiratory insufficiency. In *Proceedings. 25th Annual Conference on Engineering in Medicine and Biology*, Bal Harbour, Florida, 1–5 October 1972.
4. Lewis Thomas. 1972. Guessing and knowing: Reflections on the science and technology of medicine. *Saturday Review*, 23 December 1972, pp. 52–57.
5. Jack H.U. Brown and James F. Dickson. 1969. Instrumentation and the delivery of health services. *Science* 166:334–338.

6. *Acute Conditions: Incidence and Associated Disability. U.S. July 1967–June 1968.* National Center for Health Statistics, series 10, no. 54. Washington, D.C.: Health Services and Mental Health Administration, USPHS, HEW.
7. Morris F. Collen, chairman. 1970. *Provisional Guidelines for Automated Multiphasic Health Testing and Services.* Report of the Subcommittee on Quality Control and Operational Guidelines of the Policy Advisory Committee on AMHTS. Washington, D.C.: Health Services and Mental Health Administration, USPHS, HEW.
8. M.F. Collen, R. Feldman, A. Siegelaub, and D. Crawford. 1970. Dollar cost per positive test for automated multiphasic screening. *New Eng. J. Med.* 283:459–463.

4
National Priorities for Health and Health Care: Objectives and Criteria

Whenever the demand for goods and services greatly exceeds the available supply, their distribution or allocation to consumers must be based on some form of priorities, expressed or implied. The need for clearly defined guidelines is accentuated when government becomes intimately involved in the provision of essential needs to the general public. There is general agreement that access to high-quality health care is a *right,* not a privilege, and funds are now being dispersed for health care and health research by more than twenty federal agencies. Nevertheless no recognizable national health policy has been established, and the criteria of current national priorities must be interpreted from diverse and disparate legislative and administrative actions.

The "conquest of the leading causes of death," particularly heart disease and cancer, has become clearly established as a prime objective. In recent years legislative allocations to the National Cancer and National Heart and Lung Institutes have increased, while budgets for the institutes dealing with other problems have remained fixed or declined. By such an operational definition heart disease and cancer have attained a position of "most favored diseases," with chronic diseases of lungs and kidneys also in the forefront of recognition. The goal of conquering the major killers has a popular appeal that comes from its overtones of victory in battle or placing a man on the moon within ten years. The enormous convergence of resources on these problems has clearly provided dramatic progress, most notably including the flurry of heart transplants, the growing evidence of viruses as causes of certain cancers, the development of artificial hearts, and the rapid development of coronary-care units, now dispersed widely over the country. Such achievements clearly warrant sustaining federal support for research and clinical applications. However, it is also extremely important to consider both the health requirements that must necessarily be neglected because of this priority and the consequences of success in these health technologies.

Consequences of Technological Success

A large proportion of the most serious problems of modern society can be traced quite directly to the unpredicted results of major technological triumphs. For example, the population explosion resulted from large-scale elimination of communicable diseases and nutritional deficiencies that had historically acted to balance the very high birth rates with high death rates. The technical revolution of agriculture displaced people from the land and stimulated mass migrations to the cities, compounding the problems of metropolitan centers. The deterioration of the environment, depletion of resources, and overproduction of waste products all stem from technological accomplishments. The development of the "pill" not only helped prevent unwanted babies but also directly altered the moral and ethical values of a large segment of the population and contributed to a resurgence of venereal disease. The development of artificial vital organs, such as hearts and kidneys, constitutes a notable achievement attributable to the collaborative efforts of engineers and life scientists, but this development also presages new ethical, legal, and economic problems in the future.

Artificial kidneys were initially developed as a method of supplementing kidney function for patients suffering transient acute kidney failure but expected to recover spontaneously in a few days or weeks. It was almost inevitable that the utilization of artificial kidneys would be extended over longer periods of time, and this was made possible by a chronic arteriovenous shunt developed by Belding Scribner. During the past decade the lives of hundreds of patients have been prolonged through periodic hemodialysis several times weekly over periods of years. Many of them carry out these sophisticated procedures at home.[1] The widespread appeal of such technologies as a means of rescuing people from certain death and restoring relatively normal existence is almost irresistible. As a consequence Congress passed Social Security Amendments in 1972 (PL 92-603) which provided financial support under Medicare for workers and dependents considered disabled from chronic renal disease and expected to derive benefit from hemodialysis or kidney transplantation. Unlike the usual Medicare eligibility requirements this provision would cover nearly everyone in the country with advanced chronic renal disease. It was anticipated that 8,000 to 10,000 patients would be eligible for this sophisticated treatment during the first year and that the number would reach a stable level of about 60,000 by the tenth year. From the medical standpoint hemodialysis and kidney transplants are very effective as life-extending procedures. By the criteria described in Chapter 3 the benefits must be considered excellent and costs extremely great. The legislation became effective in July 1973, and the estimated cost for the first year was $135 million. The annual expenditures are expected to increase to about $1 billion by the tenth year, when the number of patients entering the program will approximately equal the death rate of those in the program.

A panel appointed to consider the implications of a categorical catastrophic-disease approach to National Health Insurance reported back to the National Academy of Medicine that the complete coverage of discrete categories of catastrophic diseases on a universal-eligibility basis was an unrealistic goal for the foreseeable future.[2] Among the considerations leading to this conclusion was a bill introduced to cover the treatment of some 25,000 patients with hemophilia, a disease which requires extensive medical care costing an average of $6,000 per year. The estimated annual expenditure would be about $150 million. The United States is a rich country, and its citizens are in general loath to consider depriving people of their right to survival for lack of personnel, equipment, or facilities. However, the panel expressed concern that sequential federal coverage of diseases requiring very large expenditures for each patient would lead to serious imbalance in the allocation of funds, personnel, and facilities. A compelling argument stemmed from the potential impact of future success in developing an implantable artificial heart.

The original impetus to develop artificial supplements or substitutes for heart and lung function was directed toward temporary use in specific instances. For example, artificial heart-assist devices were developed to support the lives of patients with acute myocardial infarctions during critical periods until sufficient healing and reduction in irritability of the heart muscle had occurred to allow the patient to survive on his own. In addition heart-lung machines were designed and developed to allow surgeons to repair or correct defects in the walls and valves of the heart under direct vision, a most notable achievement indeed. The stage was then set for a series of spectacular heart transplants, which captured the imagination of the public in this country and abroad. This effort has now been almost completely abandoned, at least for the present. This sequence represents an intriguing example of a major research-and-development program that was discontinued because the cost/benefit ratio was not sufficiently favorable. Not only were the financial costs extremely great (ranging as high as $65,000 for the first two weeks of care); other costs in suffering and anguish also acted as powerful negative influences.

The obvious "next step" in artificial-heart research was a major effort to develop a mechanical heart that could be installed within the chest to completely replace a heart that had been rendered incompetent by coronary atherosclerosis or myocardial infarction and that would not be subject to the rejection problem that had plagued the transplants. In 1964 the Artificial Heart Program was established by a line item in the budget as a national effort organized to support a variety of therapeutically safe and reliable cardiac-assist and total-replacement systems.[3] The original concept was based on estimates that over 100,000 persons under 65 years of age and some 250,000 over 65 die yearly from heart disease without other complications. The program was thus conceived as having to meet an ultimate demand for 200,000 implantable artificial hearts per year. The Institute of Medicine panel, mentioned above, took a much more conservative view and estimated that the number of artificial implants might range between 17,000 and 50,000 at a cost of about $35,000 for each nuclear-powered heart. If the patient load proved to be 50,000, then the annual cost would exceed $1,750,000,000, assuming no complications and no need for continuing medical care.

Although the very large economic costs are impressive and easy to quote, they are far from the most important issue. The most significant deterrent to the wholesale implantation or widespread utilization of artificial organs are the socioeconomic, legal, ethical, and philosophical implications. For example, a world threatened by a population explosion, congestion, environmental deterioration, dwindling resources, and the neglectful warehousing of senior citizens provides no encouragement for extending the lives of thousands of elderly people. As one result of such considerations a portion of the funding allocated for the Artificial Heart Program has been utilized to support research and development on improved facilities for the treatment of patients with acute heart attacks.

Coronary-care units for intensive management of patients with acute myocardial infarction have sprung up in large numbers all across the nation. Even small hospitals with relatively infrequent calls for intensive coronary care have responded to the wave of enthusiasm by installing these facilities, often at extremely great expense and questionable efficiency. It is generally acknowledged that such highly specialized services really require a relatively continuous flow of patients to maintain both efficiency and effectiveness. For example, Bernard Bloom and Osler Peterson[4] analyzed the distribution of coronary-care units in the state of Massachusetts based on certain assumptions regarding access, size, patient flow, and travel time (using a maximum of 30 minutes) and concluded that the state's 5.9 million people could be better served by 39 coronary-care units with 336 beds instead of the present 94 units with 446 beds.

Such critical evaluations of health-care services are extremely rare, despite their obvious importance in insuring a realistic allocation of resources. A unique controlled study on the relative effectiveness of coronary-care units was carried out by a group of physicians as a cooperative study in England.[5] A comparison was made between home care by the family doctor and hospital treatment in an intensive-care unit by randomly allocating 343 patients into the two groups. They found "no significant difference between the two random groups with regard to any of the characteristics recorded." There was some bias in the selection of patients since the number of patients with low blood pressure turned out to be somewhat higher in the hospital group. However, the lack of a clear advantage in clinical results from admitting patients to intensive care in hospitals is not only surprising but warrants further study. There is growing evidence that the patients who are commonly cited as having been "saved" are those who suffered hazardous cardiac arrhythmias that could be promptly treated (e.g., by defibrillation). There is also growing awareness that a substantial proportion of such patients suddenly drop dead during the subsequent year. There is thus an urgent need for a realistic evaluation of the ultimate results of such sophisticated health-care management so that sensible decisions and priorities can be based on reliable data and calm judgments, rather than on emotional considerations or professional status. Emotionally charged situations are particularly prone to unreasoned excesses, as is exemplified by life-sustaining efforts at the death bed.

Heroic Life Support of the Terminally Ill
Physicians are dedicated to the preservation of the lives of their patients to the best of their ability as an expression of the highest medical priority.

This goal was conceived at a time when physicians were essentially powerless to extend the lives of patients during terminal illness. Today virtually any hospital is fully capable of prolonging the lives of many patients through artificial substitutes for various organ functions. Robert Williams[6] has described an all too common case of a man 85 years of age with cancer, severe trauma with deep coma, and paralysis of all extremities who was kept alive by a combination of an artificial respirator, an artificial kidney, and a pacemaker (Figure 4.1A). This is an extreme example, but it contains the essence of an extremely serious problem.

There is no denying that the rapid progress in sophisticated technologies has brought very great benefits, particularly to the relatively few who need them, but these are blessings that are heavily mixed with potential anguish on the part of the patients and their families. It is time to realize that there are many occasions when death provides relief and when death with dignity becomes a highly treasured objective.

Even more crucial is the basic question of what other alternative approaches to health care are being neglected for lack of resources. There are thousands of ways that the health of citizens and the quality of their lives can be enhanced by methods that are fully developed but largely unavailable. To cite a specific example, consider the case of Dean Anderson, who was born with spina bifida and hydrocephalus (*Seattle Times*, June 20, 1974). The spinal defect was closed and hydrocephalus arrested by surgery, but he remained paralyzed from the waist down. Being considered "a hopeless case," he was installed in one of those special state repositories for 21 of his first 26 years. He is a prime example of the sequestered individual who is diverted from the mainstream of life through a one-way trapdoor, as illustrated in Figure 2.3. With the help of a friend he extricated himself from this dismal situation, attended business school, and is now employed at Northwest Bell Telephone Company typing service orders into a computer and "earning everything he's got" (Figure 4.1B). Here is a man who is self-sufficient and living a rewarding life while many individuals with lesser physical handicaps are relegated to warehouses for "surplus people." A critical evaluation of our priorities might very well shift some of our emphasis and resources toward greatly expanding the number of physically handicapped who can become more self-sufficient. The humanitarian aspects alone would warrant such an

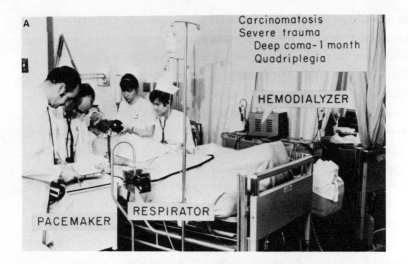

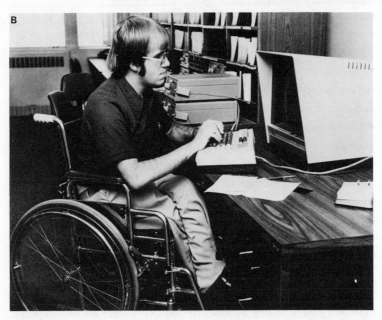

Figure 4.1 Modern technologies permit prolongation of the lives of the terminally ill beyond reasonable limits in accordance with long-established tradition and legal requirements (A). In contrast, of the millions of individuals with varying degrees of handicap languishing in institutions, only a determined few overcome the obstacles barring the way to the attainment of self-sufficiency (B). These two examples exaggerate the distinction between preservation of life at any cost and improving the quality of life as prime goals of health care.

effort, but the investment would also be financially sound in that it would allow many present tax-consumers to become self-supporting taxpayers. (Many alternatives will be presented in Chapter 7 to illustrate technologies that could make this shift in priorities both practical and rewarding.)

It seems inevitable that our new, sophisticated health technologies will require a major revision of the basic objectives of physicians and their colleagues in the health-care delivery system. In place of the single guiding principle of "saving lives" the objectives of health care may need to be broadened to include: (1) preservation of life, (2) avoidance or prevention of suffering, and (3) optimization of the quality of life and living.

Alternative Criteria for Health Priorities

Current priorities bias health-care efforts toward the older age groups. For example, Harvey Geller[7] tabulated the most probable causes of death during subsequent ten-year periods for each five-year increment of age from 5 to 70 of white and black males and females. Some representative lists showing the 12 to 16 most common diseases by age for white males are presented in Table 4.1. Comparative lists for ages 20 and 50 of black males and females are found in Table 4.2. Young people as a whole are so extremely healthy that accidents, suicides, and homicides are among the major threats to health and life during childhood, adolescence, and early adulthood. The most prevalent causes of death of individuals over 45 conform quite accurately to the present priorities for health-care research and delivery, but the chief hazards to life and health of young people are very different.

Minimizing Loss of Productive Life Span

The life expectancy of the younger age groups and the potential duration of productive life of young people is so great that a very substantial investment in the management of threats to their life and limb is warranted. The essential ingredient for the successful management of the results of accidents and violence is an effective emergency system. It is a tragedy and a disgrace that the management of emergencies is one of the weakest segments of the health-care delivery system of this country. In a

Table 4.1
Leading Causes of Death in White Males at Various Ages

Rank	Cause of Death	Chance in 100,000 of the Individual Dying from This Cause
Age 10		
1	Motor-vehicle accidents	316
2	Drowning	69
3	Accidents due to firearms	40
4	Suicide	36
5	Leukemia and aleukemia	28
6	Congenital malformation of the circulatory system	23
7	Homicide	21
8	Pneumonia	20
9	Lymphosarcoma	18
10	Accidental falls	11
11	Malignant neoplasm of brain, other nervous system parts	11
12	Water-transport accidents	9
13	Accidents due to electricity	9
14	Railway accidents	3
	Other causes	265
	Total	880
Age 20		
1	Motor-vehicle accidents	581
2	Suicide	126
3	Homicide	63
4	Drowning	40
5	Aircraft accidents	39
6	Lymphosarcoma	39
7	Nephritis and nephrosis	32
8	Water-transport accidents	32
9	Accidents due to firearms	32
10	Pneumonia	32
11	Arterioscler, heart disease and chronic endocarditis	31
12	Leukemia and aleukemia	23
13	Chronic rheumatic heart disease	23
14	Congenital malformation of the circulatory system	16
	Other causes	472
	Total	1,580

Table 4.1 (continued)
Leading Causes of Death in White Males at Various Ages

Rank	Cause of Death	Chance in 100,000 of the Individual Dying from This Cause
Age 30		
1	Arterioscler. heart disease and chronic endocarditis	329
2	Motor-vehicle accidents	302
3	Suicide	178
4	Cirrhosis of the liver	68
5	Chronic rheumatic heart disease	64
6	Vascular lesions affecting the central nervous system	55
7	Homicide	51
8	Lymphosarcoma	42
9	Nephritis and nephrosis	42
10	Pneumonia	42
11	Diabetes mellitus	42
12	Malignant neoplasm of lungs	34
13	Aircraft accidents	30
	Other causes	840
	Total	2,120
Age 40		
1	Arterioscler. heart disease and chronic endocarditis	1,877
2	Motor-vehicle accidents	285
3	Suicide	264
4	Cirrhosis of the liver	222
5	Vascular lesions affecting the central nervous system	222
6	Malignant neoplasm of lungs	202
7	Chronic rheumatic heart disease	167
8	Pneumonia	111
9	Malignant neoplasm of intestines and rectum	111
10	Other diseases of the heart	76
11	Lymphosarcoma	76
12	Malignant neoplasm of stomach and esophagus	56
13	Hypertensive heart disease	56
14	Tuberculosis	56
	Other causes	1,744
	Total	5,560

Table 4.1 (continued)
Leading Cause of Death in White Males at Various Ages

Rank	Cause of Death	Chance in 100,000 of the Individual Dying from This Cause
Age 50		
1	Arterioscler. heart disease and chronic endocarditis	5,764
2	Malignant neoplasm of lungs	860
3	Vascular lesions affecting the central nervous system	717
4	Cirrhosis of the liver	488
5	Suicide	345
6	Motor-vehicle accidents	345
7	Malignant neoplasm of intestines and rectum	287
8	Pneumonia	287
9	Chronic rheumatic heart disease	287
10	Malignant neoplasm of stomach and esophagus	287
11	Hypertensive heart disease	287
12	Other diseases of the heart	287
13	Diseases of arteries	143
14	Diabetes mellitus	143
	Other causes	3,756
	Total	14,340
Age 60		
1	Arterioscler. heart disease and endocarditis	12,697
2	Vascular lesions affecting the central nervous system	2,569
3	Malignant neoplasm of lungs	1,700
4	Malignant neoplasm of intestines and rectum	943
5	Hypertensive heart disease	813
6	Pneumonia	628
7	Malignant neoplasm of stomach and esophagus	628
8	Diseases of arteries	628
9	Cirrhosis of the liver	628
10	Other myocardial degeneration	628
11	Emphysema	628
12	Malignant neoplasm of prostate	499
13	Diabetes mellitus	499
14	Suicide	314
15	Other diseases of the heart	314
16	Motor-vehicle accidents	314
	Other causes	6,986
	Total	31,420

Table 4.2
Leading Causes of Death in Females and Black Males at Various Ages

Rank	Cause of Death	Chance in 100,000 of the Individual Dying from This Cause
White Female: Age 20		
1	Motor-vehicle accidents	119
2	Suicide	40
3	Chronic rheumatic heart disease	27
4	Vascular lesions affecting the central nervous system	23
5	Lymphosarcoma	20
6	Nephritis and nephrosis	20
7	Homicide	20
8	Pneumonia	20
9	Congenital malformation of the circulatory system	16
10	Leukemia and aleukemia	13
11	Diabetes mellitus	13
12	Malignant neoplasm of brain, other nervous system parts	10
	Other causes	319
	Total	660
White Female: Age 50		
1	Arterioscler. heart disease and chronic endocarditis	1,313
2	Malignant neoplasm of breast	631
3	Vascular lesions affecting the central nervous system	548
4	Malignant neoplasm of intestines and rectum	343
5	Malignant neoplasm of uterus	302
6	Hypertensive heart disease	246
7	Chronic rheumatic heart disease	233
8	Cirrhosis of the liver	192
9	Diabetes mellitus	178
10	Malignant neoplasm of lungs	137
11	Pneumonia	137
12	Motor-vehicle accidents	137
13	Malignant neoplasm of stomach and esophagus	109
14	Lymphosarcoma	109
15	Suicide	96
	Other causes	2,139
	Total	6,850

Table 4.2 (continued)
Leading Causes of Death in Females and Black Males at Various Ages

Rank	Cause of Death	Chance in 100,000 of the Individual Dying from This Cause
Black Female: Age 20		
1	Homicide	206
2	Motor-vehicle accidents	123
3	Vascular lesions affecting the central nervous system	95
4	Pneumonia	77
5	Tuberculosis	72
6	Chronic rheumatic heart disease	61
7	Arterioscler. heart disease and chronic endocarditis	47
8	Nephritis and nephrosis	36
9	Accidents caused by fire and explosion	32
10	Hypertensive heart disease	29
11	Cirrhosis of the liver	29
12	Suicide	18
	Other causes	985
	Total	1,810
Black Female: Age 50		
1	Arterioscler. heart disease and chronic endocarditis	2,899
2	Vascular lesions affecting the central nervous system	2,641
3	Hypertensive heart disease	1,893
4	Diabetes mellitus	748
5	Malignant neoplasm of uterus	724
6	Malignant neoplasm of breast	561
7	Other myocardial degeneration	421
8	Malignant neoplasm of intestines and rectum	421
9	Pneumonia	397
10	Other diseases of the heart	327
11	Nephritis and nephrosis	327
12	Malignant neoplasm of stomach and esophagus	327
13	Other hypertensive diseases	234
14	Cirrhosis of the liver	234
15	Infection of kidney	164
16	Diseases of arteries	164
	Other causes	3,878
	Total	16,360

Table 4.2 (continued)
Leading Causes of Death in Females and Black Males at Various Ages

Rank	Cause of Death	Chance in 100,000 of the Individual Dying from This Cause
Black Male: Age 20		
1	Homicide	803
2	Motor-vehicle accidents	611
3	Drowning	135
4	Suicide	98
5	Pneumonia	81
6	Vascular lesions affecting the central nervous system	63
7	Nephritis and nephrosis	63
8	Accidents caused by fire and explosion	63
9	Arterioscler. heart disease and chronic endocarditis	49
10	Tuberculosis	49
11	Chronic rheumatic heart disease	49
12	Accidents caused by firearms	45
	Other causes	1,031
	Total	3,140
Black Male: Age 50		
1	Arterioscler. heart disease and chronic endocarditis	4,608
2	Vascular lesions affecting the central nervous system	2,644
3	Hypertensive heart disease	1,650
4	Malignant neoplasm of lungs	995
5	Pneumonia	873
6	Malignant neoplasm of stomach and esophagus	655
7	Other diseases of the heart	655
8	Tuberculosis	436
9	Other myocardial degeneration	436
10	Motor-vehicle accidents	436
11	Diabetes mellitus	436
12	Malignant neoplasm of intestines and rectum	340
13	Homicide	314
14	Cirrhosis of the liver	314
15	Nephritis and nephrosis	314
16	Other hypertensive diseases	314
	Other causes	6,398
	Total	21,820

very real sense our failure to make adequate provision for emergency care is a direct threat to the life, life expectancy, and future of our most precious resource, namely the young people of this country.

Greatest Good for the Greatest Number

Health priorities are commonly based on mortality figures because these are the easiest statistics to collect. This leads to the placement of prime emphasis on the hazards to life and a de-emphasis of serious debilitating diseases that may destroy the quality of life without shortening it. As indicated in the preceding chapter, the means of estimating the relative value or importance of various aspects of health care and its results are extremely tenuous. For example, there is no obvious basis for judging the relative merits of allocating resources for such diverse goals as extending the lives of people with cancer, alleviating the suffering of individuals with pain syndromes, or providing needed food, glasses, and hearing aids to disadvantaged children. It is quite certain that present priorities are oriented toward the management of life-threatening ailments (see Figure 1.3). Another basis for evaluation might be an estimate of the cost/benefit ratio or the value-added.

The Cost/Benefit Ratio of, and Value Added by, Current Health-Care Approaches

The kinds of contribution made to health and well-being by various levels of health care were discussed in the preceding chapter. Although diagnosis and supportive care undoubtedly have great value to the patient, the most important consideration must ultimately be the therapeutic effectiveness of the health management. Ideally the highest level of therapeutic effectiveness is represented by the prevention, elimination, or suppression of the cause of the ailment through the direct action of health professionals. Unfortunately the number of common diseases for which such effective treatment is currently available remains rather small, certainly much smaller than most people realize. For this reason there is need to consider also the common ailments for which management can be greatly improved through better utilization of current knowledge, technologies, and facilities.

Urgent Needs for Various Levels of Disability

The various levels of disability (see Figure 2.5) will call for different essential components of the ideal health-care system. A qualitative indication of the urgent needs for some of these essential ingredients is presented in Figure 4.2. This schematic illustration indicates the obvious fact that our preoccupation with hospitals and doctors' offices as the primary sites of care have caused us to neglect seriously many other important approaches to health care. The remainder of this chapter is devoted to the identification of some neglected opportunities that should be recognized in our long-range national health priorities. Subsequent chapters will deal with a wide assortment of options by which some of these unmet needs can be more effectively covered.

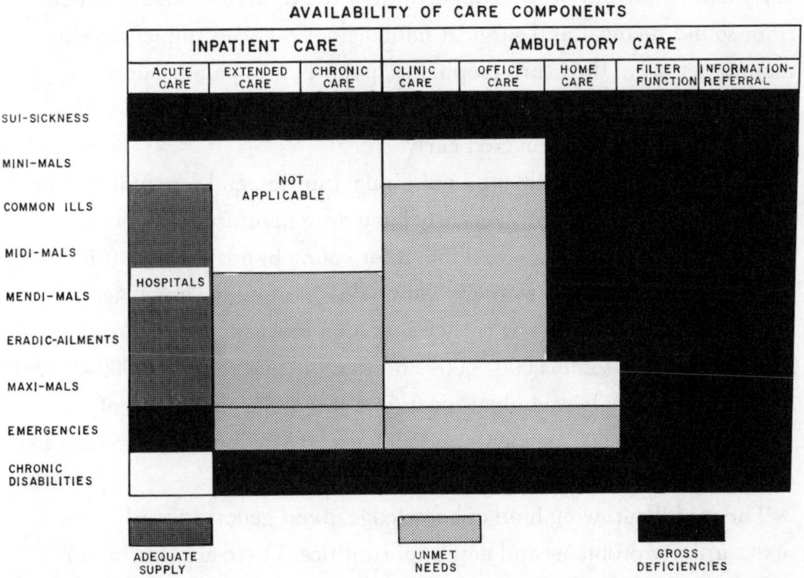

Figure 4.2 Hospital beds for the acute care of various levels of illness are available in surplus in most urban areas. Virtually all other mechanisms for management have serious unmet needs or gross deficiencies, particularly the emergency services and mechanisms for the care of chronic disabilities. Expansion of ambulatory outpatient care must involve, not only more clinic and office practice, but greater utilization of home care, self-care, screening (filter function), and effective information and referral services.

Neglected Opportunities for Infants and Children

The greatest contribution to human longevity would result from successful avoidance or treatment of the many hazards that threaten the lives of newborn babies. The period immediately after birth is fraught with both transient and longer-lasting complications, including prematurity, depression from anesthesia, birth injuries, congenital defects and deformities, and hyaline-membrane disease. Prenatal care and maternal nutrition during pregnancy are also critical. In many instances prompt and effective treatment can convert imminent tragedy into normal development, full potential, and long life. Inadequate responses can easily produce tragic and costly results. Additional hazards appear or develop in early childhood and provide opportunities to attain near-maximal benefit from sound medical and surgical management. For example, developmental defects in the heart, esophagus, pylorus, and palate can be corrected surgically. Hydrocephalus can be treated with a surgically placed shunt if it is discovered early.

Children die from accidental poisoning, injuries, and parental violence in shocking numbers. Only recently have drug manufacturers begun installing bottle caps that are difficult for young hands to open. It is impossible to estimate how many young deaths and how much agony could have been avoided by earlier action on this issue alone. Consider also the fact that some 3,000–4,000 children die and some 150,000–250,000 are injured yearly because manufacturers still make clothes out of flammable material. Accidents and violence are major threats to the safety of thousands of children.

The rapidly growing fund of knowledge about genetic disturbances opens up new problems and new opportunities. There are four broad classes of genetic disease. Major disturbances of the genes can produce complex developmental abnormalities such as Down's syndrome (otherwise known as mongolism). Abnormalities of single genes produce conditions such as hemophilia, sickle-cell anemia, and polycystic kidneys. Immunological incompatibility is represented by the well-known Rh factor. Finally, there are suspected genetic elements in common diseases such as atherosclerosis, arthritis, and diabetes. There is a need for further development of techniques such as amniocentesis for the determination of the health of fetuses in order to prepare parents and health-care personnel for such potential defects.

The number of Americans who are mentally retarded is not accurately known, but it is estimated at about 6 million (about 3% of the population). Some 80–90% of retarded youngsters could be trained up to about the sixth-grade level, but only about half are now receiving such training. The total problem is, however, not confined to the patient. The entire family is affected, particularly other children. This raises serious economic and emotional problems, especially since there are clearly established links between retardation and socioeconomic deprivation. Today more than 200,000 retarded people reside in state institutions, most of which provide grossly inadequate education or rehabilitation. The vocational training of such youngsters might prove to be, not only more kind and humane, but actually cheaper in the long run.

The prevalence of impairments that interfere with educational and social interaction in children is so very great that they seem to deserve far greater attention and effort than they are presently receiving. For example, U.S. Public Health Service statistics for the year beginning July 1968 presented data supporting the following estimates among children under 15 years for the United States as a whole: visual impairment, 328,000; hearing impairment, 467,000; speech impairment, 546,000; orthopedic defects, 1,260,000.[8] It is manifestly impractical to undertake comprehensive screening programs to elicit all possible ailments of children. Mothers are in a position to observe their children better than anyone else, but they are generally not fully informed of the critical signs and symptoms, or of their significance.

A useful example is the problem of deafness or hearing loss in young children. Many children suffer a hearing loss at birth or shortly thereafter that remains undetected. Often the child is regarded as "slow" or "retarded." If a severe hearing defect goes unrecognized during the first two years of life when the central nervous connections for speech are being developed, correcting the deafness with a hearing aid will still leave a severe residual speech defect. Such children require long and patient training to teach them to understand the spoken word and to speak intelligibly. Every mother should be made aware of a few simple tests that can elicit evidence of deafness as a part of prenatal management.[9]

Although many health problems can be cured or effectively treated, others present persistent difficulties that require rehabilitation if the affected children are to approach their full potential (Figure 4.3). Unfortunately the economic significance of investing capital to provide greater independence and self-sufficiency to physically handicapped children has never been analyzed.

Fortunately it is not necessary to choose between providing health care for the "most favored illnesses" and treating the diseases of infants and children. The resources currently allocated to medical research, health personnel, facilities, and rehabilitation for our youth can and should be greatly increased, preferably on the basis of sound planning.

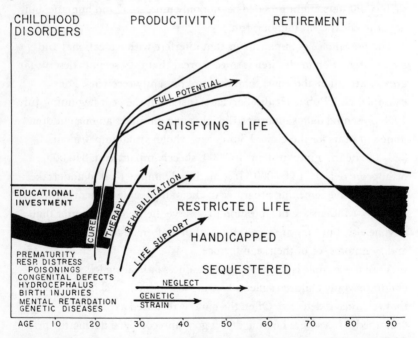

Figure 4.3 The successful management of childhood disorders includes assuring appropriate educational investment, therapeutic rehabilitation, and life support to provide the maximum opportunities for a productive and satisfying life. The denial of opportunities to children leads to a restricted life, physical handicaps, and a sequestered existence. The costs of early and effective therapy must be weighed against the waste of human potential and the expense of long-term maintenance and chronic care.

Health Needs for Youths and Young Adults

Society has a heavy responsibility to preserve and restore health to men and women during the productive periods of their lives, particularly those who have family responsibilities. Incapacitation of either parent can have serious and lasting effects on the entire family unit. For this reason attention must be directed toward the provisions that should be available to take care of their most common and pressing needs.

Violence, Trauma, and Emergencies

Safety experts estimate that 1.9 million people have died in motor-vehicle accidents—almost twice the number killed in all of our wars. This figure neglects the millions who have been injured, hospitalized, or incapacitated. Automobiles have been so heavily indicted that we tend to lose sight of the fact that the largest number of accidents occurs in the home.[10] The appalling toll of persons killed and injured by accidents along with the pain, suffering, economic losses, and annual costs of accidents and accidental injuries are summarized in Table 4.3 for 1965 (see also Figure 4.4).

What are our provisions for the care of accident victims? A committee of the National Research Council has reported that emergency services represent "one of the weakest links in the delivery of health care in the nation." [11] Accidental trauma represents the "leading killer of Americans between the ages of 1 and 38 years" and is *the* neglected disease of modern society. It was estimated that as many as 18% of automobile fatalities could have been averted if the victims had received proper emergency treatment. The United States has developed the most extensive network of sophisticated communications and transportation systems conceivable, but this enormous capacity is not being utilized in support of emergency services. In most parts of the country ambulances are not equipped with radios or any other communication link to medical advice. The drivers and attendants are inadequately trained, and a majority of the ambulances are owned and operated by mortuaries. Most emergency rooms in hospitals are served on a part-time basis or by interns and residents. Ambulance drivers are often inadequately informed about the capabilities of the emergency rooms they approach. In short the most

Table 4.3

Major Facts about Accidental Injuries and Deaths, 1965

Persons killed	104 thousand
Persons killed by motor vehicles	46 thousand
Persons injured	52 million
Persons injured by moving motor vehicles	over 3 million
Persons bed-disabled by injury	11 million
Persons receiving medical care for injuries	45 million
Persons hospitalized by injuries	2 million
Days of restricted activity	512 million
Days of bed-disability	132 million
Days of work loss	90 million
Days of school loss	11 million
Hospital bed-days	22 million
Hospital beds required for treatment	65 thousand
Hospital personnel required for treatment	88 thousand
Annual cost of accidents	$16 billion
Annual cost of accidental injuries	$10 billion

It is estimated that the prevalence of physical impairments caused by injuries in the noninstitutionalized population of the United States is over 11 million. Source: Epidemiology and Surveillance Branch, Division of Accident Prevention, January 20, 1966.

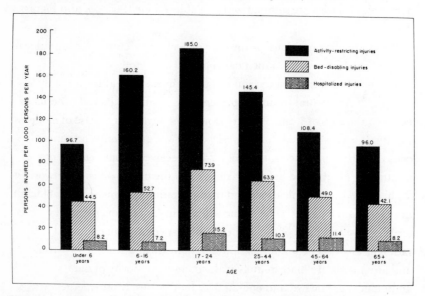

Figure 4.4 A large number of Americans have suffered serious injuries that restrict their activity (black areas), confine them to bed (crosshatched areas), or require hospitalization (herringbone-patterned areas). The incidence is high in all age groups but is greatest in ages 17–24 years. From *Persons Injured and Disability Days Due to Injury*.[10]

essential requirements for supporting the health and futures of young people are being neglected. Clearly a reassessment of priorities is sorely needed. In the past few years the problem has become more widely appreciated, and initial steps of importance are being taken. (Some alternatives and approaches to emergency care will be considered in subsequent chapters.)

Further strides could be made by improving the safety of automobiles. For example, Nicholas Perrone[12] estimates that, if the energy-absorbing properties of vehicles were increased through the addition of about 200 pounds to a car, the return on investment would be about 20:1. He concluded that "safety pays for itself." Unfortunately we have been "penny wise and pound foolish" in our priorities.

Geographic Gaps in Health Care

Health-care delivery unexcelled anywhere in the world is readily available to people fortunate enough to live in the more affluent sections of metropolitan and suburban areas in this country. There is a super-abundance of fine hospitals, well-trained physicians, and other health professionals using the most sophisticated technologies. Indeed there is a recognized surplus of physicians and of hospital beds in these areas, while other parts of the country suffer serious deficiencies in all necessary elements of health-care delivery. In the ghettos of central cities a few physicians serve large numbers of disadvantaged people whose health needs are greatly exacerbated by their undesirable socioeconomic condition. The allocation of additional money for Medicare and Medicaid will not solve this complex problem because these programs do not focus on the root issues. We have failed to develop the incentives necessary to distribute the surplus resources of health-care personnel and facilities more equitably among people so close geographically and yet so distant in terms of their environmental conditions (see also Figures 5.5. and 5.6).

The people who live in rural areas also commonly suffer from insufficient access to good health care. Many counties are without a single physician, so that they must depend upon distant towns and cities for their health care. Inadequate access to health care is a sorry enough condition for those rural people who can afford to pay; the plight of poor farmers and migrant workers is even more tragic than that of the ghetto dwellers because geographic isolation compounds their socioeconomic disadvantages.

The people who inhabit remote areas of the country, far from the nearest settlement, must either develop a high level of self-reliance in managing illness or be prepared to travel long distances to medical centers. In remote areas of Alaska, the mountain states, the southwest, and elsewhere the necessary communications and transportation resources have not been mobilized despite the fact that these technologies are fully developed and could be made readily available without further time lags. Some alternatives for this process will be discussed in Chapter 5.

Unmet Needs for Different Races

We have heard much about the inadequate health care afforded black Americans, while equally severe deficiencies are faced by Puerto Ricans, Chicanos, Filipinos, Orientals, and others. By any standard, however, it is the native American who suffers most from the inadequacy and unavailability of health resources, despite the efforts of the Indian Health Service, which is responsible to some 400,000 American Indians and Alaskan natives.

The infant mortality rate of native Americans is more than three times that of whites. The documentation of risk factors predisposing to illness in infants adds insight into some of the fundamental problems faced by native Americans.[13] Infants (0–12 months) are found to have a very high incidence of morbidity if they have three to five of the following risk factors: (1) low birth weight (less than six pounds), (2) respiratory distress at birth, (3) congenital defect, (4) child neglect, (5) alcoholism in one parent, (6) more than five brothers and sisters, (7) mental problems in parents, (8) overcrowded home, (9) living in a high-risk community. Note the emphasis on socioeconomic factors in this list.

American Indians are protesting against their living conditions; and the impact of their plight on their health is an important issue by any definition. Consider, for example, the comparisons shown in Table 4.4.

The crude death rate of Alaskan natives is more than twice that of white Alaskans. The four principal causes of death in the native population in

Table 4.4

	American Indian	U.S. population
Suicides (per 100,000)	32	16
Life expectancy	47 years	70.8 years
Infant mortality (per 1,000)	30.9	21.8
Unemployment rate	45% (estimated)	5.8%
Median family income	$4,000	$9,867

1966 were accidents, influenza, pneumonia, and diseases of early infancy. The death rate of natives from influenza and pneumonia was ten times that of whites, accidents three times, and suicides two times.

Respiratory infections are extremely common, and in children they frequently produce serious bronchiectasis, which is very rare among children in other parts of the country. Otitis media is also very common and produces severe hearing losses. Some 38% of native children were found to have significant hearing handicaps by age four. Such infections tend to keep young children sick a significant part of the time. The director of the Alaskan Native Medical Center has suggested that the high rate of mental retardation is largely due to the residual damage of acute infectious diseases early in life. These disgraceful conditions must be given great emphasis in any assessment of our national health priorities.

The Plight of the Mentally Ill

The pressures and stresses of modern society have led to an increasing incidence of psychological, psychoneurotic, and psychiatric disorders. Although these problems may not be accompanied by objective signs or organic disturbances, they are no less distressing to the patients and their families. More than 50% of all hospital beds are occupied by people with serious emotional or mental disorders. Expanded use of mood-altering drugs has allowed many of them to return to the community, but the ultimate results of this trend cannot yet be estimated.

The proportion of individuals in the general population who assert that they have had a "nervous breakdown" or have at some time felt like they were going to have one is quite large (it is estimated that some 5.4 million have had some degree of nervous breakdown). Unfortunately the major clinical criteria for psychological and psychiatric disturbances are so intangible that neither diagnoses nor effectiveness of therapy can be confidently estimated. This deficiency was dramatized by the experience of eight individuals who voluntarily made an appointment with different mental-hospital admissions offices and stated they "had been hearing voices" (reported in the *New York Times*, January 20, 1973). They complained of no other symptoms and gave factual histories on all other aspects of their past except for using fictitious names. Seven of these volunteers were diagnosed as schizophrenics and the eighth was classified as manic-depressive. They were admitted to mental wards for periods between 7 and 52 days before being released. Not one had the diagnosis modified and none was released as cured. All were given a final evaluation of "in remission." While in the mental hospitals they recorded nearly 1,500 instances when reasonable questions were ignored or avoided. They witnessed depersonalization and abuse.

Even without such nonconventional and overly dramatic evidence, there is ample reason to regard our management of the mentally ill as inadequate and greatly in need of more fundamental research, greater allocation of resources, and a more effective therapeutic methodology based on more objective and scientific principles. Techniques and technologies which have proved valuable in providing objective and quantitative diagnostic data for organic diseases should be more widely used by psychiatrists. The functional accompaniment of nervous tensions could provide added insight into the emotional state of individuals through measurements of variations in heart rate, sweating, respiratory activity, muscle tension, encephalographic potentials, etc. In short, a whole new era is needed in the field of mental health.

There are some experts who confidently expect that biochemical changes in the brain metabolism will emerge as a primary cause of and also as a basis of direct therapy for mental illness. Robert Williams[14] has directed attention to certain mental abnormalities that can be associated with metabolic disorders. For example, a correlation of mental changes with blood levels of calcium is noted in hyperparathyroidism. Phenylketonuria and galactosemia are also related to emotional disturbances. The Lesch-Nyhan syndrome produces retardation and compulsive self-mutilation based on a genetic enzyme disturbance. Cushing's disease and cretinism are more familiar examples of metabolic diseases with mental effects. It is thus quite possible that the future prospects for some of the mentally ill may be greatly improved by scientific breakthroughs in metabolic research.

The magnitude of the problem of institutionalization is extremely great, and its costs are so enormous that a very large investment in basic research and clinical investigation could easily be justified. Some estimates by Dorothy Rice[15] illustrate the size and scope of the problem. As of 1963 she found that almost 1.5 million people were institutionalized in mental hospitals at an estimated cost of nearly $3 billion. Some 175,000 mentally handicapped persons were institutionalized at a cost of nearly $500 million. In addition individuals in nursing homes and homes for the aged amounted to some 450,000 at an annual cost of $1.2 billion. Mechanisms that would reduce the need for such expensive institutionalization while improving the environment and quality of life for former inmates would surely justify the expense and effort. Home-based health care could be one approach (see Chapter 7). Moreover, as our society undergoes the transition from an industrial to a service orientation, the increased manpower that may be required to institute new programs for the mentally ill and the retarded will become more readily available.

Real Security for Senior Citizens

The United States is a youthful nation, and its people are preoccupied with youth to the point that the American Dream is being converted into an American Nightmare for an ever-increasing number of individuals. Many of our senior citizens labored hard and long to accumulate sufficient resources to carry them through a tranquil and pleasant retirement. They were born in a period when the older generation was held in a position of respect by a younger generation that felt a responsibility for their welfare. In their lifetimes attitudes and value systems have so changed that older Americans now tend to feel isolated, alienated, insecure, unwanted, and often seriously neglected by their offspring, who are concentrating on their own immediate interests and problems. The wisdom and experience of grandparents are no longer being passed on to youth because they are not an integral part of the family. The satisfaction of being needed, useful, and respected is largely denied them. As one consequence the suicide rate per 100,000 population at age 65 is about four times the rate at 40 years of age.

These are no small problems because we live in an era of aging populations. Since 1900 the population of the country has more than doubled, but the age group 65 and older has increased by four times. A widespread belief holds that the intellectual capacity progressively declines after the age of 50, but recent indications suggest little change in intellectual ability at least until age 60. Nevertheless the prospects of gainful employment past the age of 65 are relatively slight, even if psychological and physical requirements make this an urgent need. External contacts and stimulation are of vital importance to older people, yet many find themselves incarcerated in storage facilities to live out sad and lonesome years. There are some 30,000 such institutions, and a large proportion do an inferior job.

Unmet Needs in Anticipation of Death

Physicians consider death as something to be prevented at all costs and yet also as something to be accepted as inevitable and natural. This dichotomy of attitudes leads to difficult moral questions when technology provides opportunities to support life with heroic measures that are inconsistent with a patient's desire "to die with dignity." Dying is vastly more complicated than it used to be when most people died at home. The percent of terminally ill people in hospitals or nursing homes is placed variously between 62% and 80%. They live longer and are more likely to experience lingering death.

In the past few years widespread concern has developed regarding the process of dying and the means by which a patient can be provided with needed sympathy and support along the way.[16] Among the most articulate writers on the subject is Elisabeth Kubler-Ross,[17] who has described five stages in the process of dying: (1) denial of the prospect and hope for survival, (2) anger, (3) bargaining, (4) depression, and (5) acceptance of the inevitable.

Today's patients may not be permitted to die in peace, but they are extremely likely to die in ignorance since most health professionals find it difficult, if not impossible, to discuss the problems of dying with patients. A majority of physicians are opposed for various reasons to telling a patient that his illness is probably terminal, but indications are that it is the physician who is usually least able to face up to the fact. In most hospitals patients suspecting they may be facing death are unable to find anyone who will break the conspiracy of silence.

Organizations devoted to spreading the concept of "natural death" have sprouted—an approach comparable to the current trend toward natural childbirth. A new medical specialty called *thanotology* has sprung up for the purpose of learning more about the problems and proper treatment of terminal patients. These are sensitive issues which have rarely been openly discussed, and our knowledge about them is correspondingly sparse. Here again we are forced to face up to the consequences of our technological successes by identifying newly created problems, exploring them, and coming up with innovative solutions. For example, there is some evidence that, when patients find someone who understands and is willing to talk about their imminent death, their pain becomes more bearable, as indicated by a diminished need for medication.

These problems are of such recent vintage that our most advanced efforts are primitive and groping. Of the 7,000 hospitals in this country there may be 70 with active programs to aid dying patients. There is a real need for interdisciplinary participation involving religion, ethics, philosophy, and law. For example, the Euthanasia Educational Fund has distributed more than 50,000 copies of a "living will" addressed to the patient's family, physician, clergyman, and lawyer asking that he not be kept alive by artificial or heroic means if there is no reasonable expectation of recovery. The legal status of such documents is at the moment highly questionable, but the concept points the way to a more open and positive approach to death.

Summary

The present priorities for health are based on the "atomic-age" premise that a mobilization of sufficient resources will conquer the most important diseases affecting the population. With an aging population and with power vested in people of older ages, emphasis has been focused mainly on the "big killers" such as cancer and cardiovascular disease. Other diseases, such as sickle-cell anemia, cystic fibrosis, etc., have attained the most-favored status for various reasons but without obvious regard for the state of knowledge or the prospects for cure or prevention.

The resources available for research and development need to be extended to cover the health problems of other, broader segments of the population. For example, injuries due to accidents and violence are by far the most common threats to health among the youth and young adults of this country, while the emergency services expected to deal with these problems are among the weakest features of American health care. The potential rewards of directing effort toward the recognition, prevention, and management of illnesses of the very young are very great because they offer improved prospects for full and productive lifetimes. The deficiencies in health care available to certain groups (e.g., native Americans) are tragic and shameful. These aspects of the system, at least, deserve major overhaul. A far more realistic and sensitive approach to illness among senior citizens and patients in terminal illness is required, particularly with a progressively aging population.

All these considerations lead to a greatly broadened view of the priorities for health care that need to be established in our long-range planning. Sample options and attractive alternatives for attaining some of these goals are summarized in each of the following chapters.

References

1. C.R. Blagg, R.O. Kickman, J.W. Eschback, and B.H. Scribner. 1970. Home hemodialysis: Six years experience. *New Eng. J. Med.* 283:1126–1128.
2. H.M. Somers, chairman. 1973. *Disease by Disease Toward National Health Insurance.* Report of a Panel on the Implications of a Categorical Catastrophic Disease Approach to National Health Insurance. Washington, D.C.: Institute of Medicine, National Academy of Sciences.
3. F.W. Hastings and L.J. Marmison. 1969. *Proceedings. National Heart Institute Artificial Heart Program Conference,* Washington, D.C., 9–13 June 1969. Washington, D.C.: U.S. Government Printing Office.
4. Bernard S. Bloom and Osler L. Peterson. 1974. Patient needs and medical care planning. *New Eng. J. Med.* 290:1171–1177.
5. H.G. Mather, N.G. Pearson, K.L.Q. Read, D.B. Shaw, G.R. Stead, M.G. Thorne, S. Jones, C.J. Guerrier, C.D. Eraut, P.M. McHugh, N.R. Chowdhury, M.H. Jafary, and T.J. Wallace. 1971. Acute myocardial infarction: Home and hospital treatment. *Brit. Med. J.* 3:334–338.
6. Robert H. Williams. 1967. Our role in the generation, modification and termination of life. *Arch. Intern. Med.* 124:215–237.
7. Harvey Geller. 1966. *Probability Study of Deaths in the Next Ten Years from Specific Causes.* Philadelphia: Jefferson Medical College.

8. *Children and Youth: Selected Health Characteristics. U.S. 1958–1968.* National Center for Health Statistics, series 10, no. 62. Washington, D.C.: Health Services and Mental Health Administration, USPHS, HEW.

9. M.P. Downs and W.G. Hemenway. 1972. Newborn screening revisited. *Hearing and Speech News*, August 1972.

10. *Persons Injured and Disability Days Due to Injury.* National Center for Health Statistics, series 10, no. 58. Washington, D.C.: Health Services and Mental Health Administration, USPHS, HEW.

11. *Social Forces and the Nation's Health.* 1968. Washington, D.C.: Health Services and Mental Health Administration, USPHS, HEW.

12. Nicholas Perrone. 1970. *A Position Paper on Vehicle Safety.* Washington, D.C.: The Catholic University of America.

13. Steven J. Englender and Charles R. Strotz. 1970. *Correlation Between Risk Factors and Subsequent Infant Morbidity.* Tucson, Ariz.: Indian Health Service, Office of Management Information Systems, Health Program Systems Center.

14. Robert H. Williams. 1969. Our role in the generation, modification and termination of life. *Arch. Intern. Med.* 124:215–237.

15. Dorothy P. Rice. 1967. Estimating the cost of illness. *Am. J. Public Health* 57:424–440.

16. Robert H. Williams, ed. 1973. *To Live, To Die: When, Where and How?* New York: Springer-Verlag.

17. Elisabeth Kubler-Ross. 1973. Life and death: Lessons from the dying. In *To Live, To Die*, ed. Robert H. Williams. New York: Springer-Verlag.

5
Health-Personnel Requirements

The widespread belief that the United States suffers from a severe shortage of physicians stems in part from a greatly increased demand for adequate health care caused by increasing affluence, widespread third-party payment mechanisms, and social legislation. The natural response to this "physician shortage" has been to increase incentives to build and expand medical schools. There are reasons to believe that merely graduating more doctors will not solve the deep-seated manpower problems of health-care delivery.

The Nature and Extent of Physician Shortages

Contrary to popular belief, the shortage of physicians in this country results more from excessive specialization and maldistribution than from insufficient numbers of health professionals. The number of family physicians is grossly inadequate for current needs, while certain categories of specialists have been trained in excess of actual requirements. These surplus physicians concentrate in metropolitan and suburban areas, while remote and rural areas suffer deficiencies of health care, many of which cannot be realistically offset merely by dispersing physicians into these areas. The physician's time is often spent in routine tasks that would be more appropriately assigned to other health professionals and para-professionals. Recognition that some apparent shortages of physicians are more realistically attributable to ineffective utilization, maldistribution, and indiscriminate specialization should lead to more attainable future remedies for current dilemmas.

Between 1963 and 1969 about 7,000 doctors graduated annually from schools of medicine,[1] totaling about 42,000 physicians for the six years. Over 31,000 of these doctors elected to engage in full-time research, hospital administration, teaching, government, or other activities, leaving only about 11,000 (25% of the total) being added to the medical manpower pool in active practice. Equally important is the fact that during this period the number of general practitioners actually diminished by about 14,000, leaving less than 55,000 total in 1969, while the number of specialists has continued to rise each year.

In the decade 1955–1965 the number of active physicians increased at a slightly higher rate than the population growth (Figure 5.1). In contrast the number of professional nurses, nonprofessional nurses, and medical auxiliary personnel increased at nearly four times that rate.[2] At the turn of the century each practicing physician was largely self-sufficient, being supported on the average by only one other person. Less than a decade ago the corresponding relationship was one physician to four health professionals, of whom two were nurses. The current ratio is 1:13, and projections indicate future ratios of 1:20 or even 1:25.[3] In other words the rapidly increasing demand for health care can be met only by a greatly increased reliance on many categories of health professionals (see Table 5.1).

The Future Role of Nurses

The total pool of trained nurses is reported to be over 500,000, not counting the large number who, for many reasons, are not working at their profession. The current progressive upgrading of the role of nurses might draw a substantial number of nurses back into active practice, for it is now being realized that nurses are a most effective source of sympathetic care and concern in all aspects of health care, and that they can function independently of doctors in many instances.

In many hospitals selected nurses have been relieved of routine tasks and awarded more responsibility. This upward shift in responsibility is but a token of the changes needed. It is, for example, frequently noted that up to one-third of the nurse's time is still spent on clerical and other routine functions. An exciting example of the potential contribution of nurses has been brought to light by recent experience in coronary-care units. When the first group of such units was set up, a great variability in patient mortality rates was noted in different institutions. It was later discovered that where specially trained nurses were given authority to proceed on their own initiative with the administration of drugs and defibrillation, the survival rate was greatly improved over that of units in which the nurses

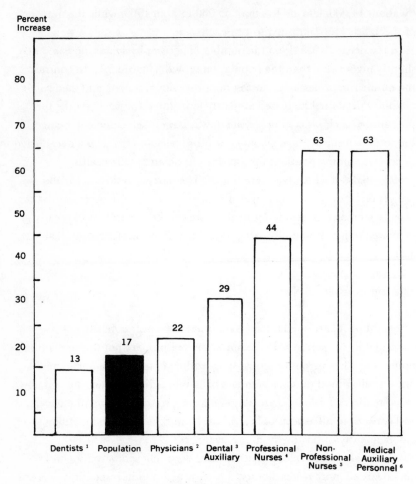

−Percentage Increases From 1955–1965 in Population and
Health Manpower

[1] Active Non-Federal Dentists.
[2] Active M.D.'s.
[3] Dental Hygienists, Assistants, and Laboratory Personnel.
[4] Active Professional Nurses.
[5] Practical Nurses, Aides, Orderlies, and Attendants.
[6] Radiologic Technologists and Clinical Laboratory Personnel.

Figure 5.1 The number of physicians in active practice increased only slightly faster than did the population during the decade 1955–1965. In contrast the number of nurses and technical support personnel increased nearly four times as rapidly. This indicates the extent to which health-care delivery has become dependent upon the full spectrum of health professionals and technicians. From the *Report of the National Advisory Commission on Health Manpower*.[8]

Table 5.1
Personnel Needs in Hospitals

		Additional Personnel Needed	
Category of Personnel	Present	Urgently	Optimum Care
Professional nurses	370,000	56,920	83,300
Licensed practical nurses	148,500	14,100	42,800
Aides, orderlies, etc.	373,100	14,200	48,700
Psychiatric aides	156,200	7,600	31,300
Medical technologists	52,900	4,100	9,100
Radiologic technicians	23,700	1,000	3,900
Laboratory assistants	14,400	800	2,400
Medical records personnel:			
Professional	6,200	600	1,800
Technical	10,000	300	1,800
Surgical technicians	17,400	500	3,800
Dieticians	12,600	1,600	3,600
Food service managers	5,300	100	800
Cytotechnologists	1,600	0	500
Histologic technicians	3,900	0	600
Electrocardiograph technicians	5,900	0	900
Electroencephalogram technicians	1,900	0	400
X-ray assistants	5,700	0	900
Occupational therapists	4,600	1,200	2,800
Occupational therapy assistants	5,600	0	1,500
Physical therapists	8,000	800	2,800
Physical therapy assistants	5,200	0	1,100
Speech pathologists and audiologists	1,000	0	600
Recreation therapists	4,600	100	1,900
Inhalation therapists	5,500	600	2,300
Pharmacists	9,500	600	1,900
Pharmacy assistants	5,500	100	900
Medical librarians	2,900	0	800
Social workers	12,100	2,000	6,400
Social work assistants	1,500	0	600
All other professional and technical	105,900	1,300	15,100
Total professional and technical	1,380,800	108,600	275,300
Food service	NA	2,600	NA
Laundry	NA	300	NA
Housekeeping	NA	2,800	NA
Maintenance	NA	2,800	NA
Management	NA	300	NA
Secretarial, clerical	NA	2,900	NA
Total other personnel	NA	11,700	NA

Source: *Social Forces and the Nation's Health*. Estimates for all registered hospitals are based on a U.S. Public Health Service–American Hospital Association survey. Columns 1 and 3 are based on 4,600 returns; column 2 is based on 421 returns. (NA = not available)

were required to obtain the approval or help of a physician for such lifesaving measures.

A project has been reported in which patients attending an ambulatory clinic (for hypertension, atherosclerotic heart disease, arthritis, obesity, etc.) were divided into two groups, with one receiving all their medical care from a nurse.[4] The result was that nurses were accepted by patients as a primary source of care, and that the improved adherence to schedules and lower cost were greatly appreciated. Nurses serving as anesthetists have been drawn into a professional void in many smaller hospitals. The development of mechanical monitoring devices that provide precise and reliable indications of a patient's condition has greatly aided in assuring a more proper utilization of nurses and others with special training. A variety of trials are under way to evaluate expanded roles for nurses in handling patients with chronic disease, including atherosclerosis, anticoagulation, diabetes, tuberculosis, and alcoholism.[5] Nurses also have a natural place in prenatal and well-baby care.[6] In most countries of Western Europe nurse-midwives assume responsibility for most normal pregnancies, including prenatal care, deliveries, and subsequent follow-up. The infant and maternal mortality rates in those countries are lower than our own, so that the American obstetrician has been called the highest-paid midwife in the world. A survey of 174 countries in 1966 reported 600,000 midwives in 153 countries, covering 75% of the world's population.[7]

Public-health nurses have a long and distinguished history of providing essential family health care in the homes of the disadvantaged. The shortage of doctors in remote and rural areas is stimulating nurse-practitioners to engage in the provision of primary care. Medical supervision of such practice is commonly supplied for legal protection, but this requirement will probably diminish, particularly in settings where other alternatives are available.

Physicians' Assistants

There has in recent years been a widely recognized need for a new member of the health-care team who would be able to perform a limited set of functions normally reserved for physicians. As of 1970 [8] some twenty different training programs for such physicians' assistants were under way around the country. These included four-year baccalaureate programs as well as programs for specialized training in such fields as children's health care, intensive care, ophthalmology, anesthesia, and emergency care.

The need for new types of physicians' assistants is growing, both in general practice and in sophisticated medical centers, and the general category is now usually broken down into three major subcategories.[9] Type-A assistants are capable of approaching the patient, collecting historical and physical data, organizing these data, and presenting them so clearly that the physician can visualize the medical problem and arrive at diagnostic and therapeutic decisions. They might be called "physicians' associates." Usually functioning under medical direction, they might act without immediate surveillance on some specific occasions. Type-B assistants are not expected to be so fully prepared with general medical knowledge; they would, however, have exceptionally detailed training in some clinical specialty, beyond that possessed by the Type-A assistant and even that of physicians not engaged in the specialty. One example may be a technician performing special functions in a renal-dialysis unit. Type-C assistants have functions similar to those of Type-A assistants, but they have less training and therefore less independence.

One important source of personnel for some of these programs might be the pool of some 6,000 medical corpsmen who leave the armed forces each year after having completed extensive coursework in basic medical sciences and having received invaluable on-the-job training and experience in hospital and outpatient settings. Until recently these military medical corpsmen were totally lost to the health professions, even if they had an interest in qualifying for civilian jobs in health care, because there was no slot in the medical establishment into which they fit. The extent to which these men can extend the services of physicians is now being actively evaluated.[10]

Diversification of Allied Health Personnel

An expanding array of personnel are now being trained to perform special kinds of functions for the benefit of patients, usually in hospital settings. A partial listing of such categories is presented in Table 5.1. These varied areas of responsibility extend from manual and menial duties to professional services in particular areas such as occupational therapy, physical therapy, speech and hearing, inhalation therapy, pharmaceutics, and social work. This impressive but incomplete array of allied health personnel highlights the limitations of the care that can be provided by a solo physician in general practice who lacks direct access to the innovations of modern medicine.

The personnel requirements listed in Table 5.1 were specifically identified in relation to *hospital* needs. The many valuable services provided by these people are not readily available to ambulatory patients or to people who might need them at home (see also Chapter 7). Unfortunately the people most in need of many of these services are senior citizens, the physically handicapped, and the disadvantaged—those who are least able to gain access to them. Enormously rewarding and satisfying careers might thus be developed for many of our unemployed and underemployed if we could create mechanisms to provide essential training in the health-related services and a framework in which these services could be dispensed to those most in need of them. The number and scope of opportunities are limited only by our willingness to reorder our priorities and mobilize the necessary resources.

Technical-Support Personnel

The progressively increasing sophistication of medical technology calls for an ever-expanding array of people capable of operating, maintaining, calibrating, and evaluating data from equipment ranging in complexity from simple diagnostic devices, x-ray machines, automated clinical chemistry machines, and multiphasic laboratories, to intensive-care units. Higher levels of competence are also required for the maintenance and repair of much of this equipment. Most hospitals are administered by managers lacking training or experience in the kind of technology so profusely distributed throughout their areas of responsibility. Hospital administrations are therefore displaying a growing interest in hiring new types of clinical engineers to translate needs into specifications, to assure compatibility of equipment, to organize repairs and preventive maintenance, and to assure safety in this maze of electronics. The newly developing career opportunities for engineers in hospitals call in turn for the development of new types of educational experiences.

As medical devices become routinized and perfected, the prior training required to operate them may well diminish. Remarkable success has been reported by Gilbert and his colleagues at the Straub Medical Research Institute of Hawaii in the planned utilization of paramedical personnel in automated health testing and appraisal.[11] Diagnostic carrels were developed for efficient acquisition of initial patient data banks, including automated histories and numerous laboratory tests. This data acquisition is accomplished routinely by "diagnostic technicians" who are high-school graduates with three to six months' training. They test hearing, vision, and pulmonary function, perform blood counts and urinalysis, take x-rays, and record electrocardiograms. With added experience some technicians have read as many as 5,000 electrocardiograms with precision. Reliability comparable to regular medical care has been attained during four years of testing and 30,000 health evaluations. Such experiences should encourage the medical community to take full advantage of opportunities to delegate increased responsibility to allied health personnel with appropriate training. By virtue of modern technology a technician with very limited training can perform 100 times as many biochemical tests with greater precision and reliability than that evidenced by the most highly trained technician only a few years ago.

Health Guides and Gatekeepers

The greatest single problem in the delivery of health care is prompt and effective entry into the system. General practitioners have traditionally served as an initial point of contact in the various countries of Western Europe and elsewhere, but the supply of general practitioners and primary-care physicians in the United States is clearly inadequate to cover this essential assignment. As a result a growing number of people descend upon emergency rooms with ailments that are not emergencies and then receive unsatisfactory management in this inappropriate setting. There is a clear need for some new and more effective mechanisms by which patients with various levels of health problems can be promptly directed to sources of information, advice, guidance, and management appropriate to their particular complaints.

An accumulating mass of experience and data suggests that the role of guide and gatekeeper for the health-care system can be effectively assumed by young and responsible people with limited special training. The number of encouraging experiments is growing. The experience at the Straub Clinic is a case in point. Another example is a systematic collaborative effort between the Beth Israel Hospital (Harvard Medical School) and the MIT Lincoln Laboratory based on the hypothesis that a significant fraction of patient-physician encounters can be safely managed by non-physicians utilizing well-defined and carefully evaluated decision trees called "protocols." [12] Nurses, physicians' assistants, or even paramedics with minimal past experience can be trained in a short time (as little as four weeks) to manage patient encounters and to refer questionable cases to a physician when so guided by a protocol.

A protocol* focuses on a specific disease or medical complaint. It indicates the appropriate history, physical examination, and laboratory data to be obtained. Once these clinical data are obtained, the protocol then includes precise rules for medical action, answering such questions as: What is the next step to be taken? What is the proper therapy? What should the patient be told? Does the patient need to be examined by a physician? The protocols include branching logic so that the data to be obtained from a given patient, and the medical actions recommended for that patient, are "individualized" according to the patient's age, sex, past history, current medications, and also according to the specific clinical data obtained from that patient. Originally an interactive computer system helped specify the order in which questions should be asked for most effective progress toward appropriate decisions and actions. As the protocols become standardized, they are evaluated and approved by medical standards and are then reduced to a relatively simple printed (not computerized) form which displays all of the necessary decision-tree logic. These forms can then be used by paramedical personnel to perform a substantial workup of the patient in advance of, and often in place of, a visit with the physician.

Previous studies have indicated that only twelve very common symptoms account for about 70% of the complaints that bring patients into

* This description was prepared by Drs. Herbert Sherman and Anthony Komaroff.

contact with physicians (see Figure 8.1). Therefore a relatively few protocols deal with a large number of patient visits. Each protocol is modified over time according to carefully monitored prospective studies, with the goal of improving diagnostic accuracy and reducing cost.

One of the first protocols developed was for symptoms of upper-respiratory infections, because of their overwhelming frequency. This protocol is displayed in Figure 5.2A. It uses color coding and symbols to represent a relatively complex decision-making scheme. The protocol format developed by the Beth Israel–Lincoln Lab group condenses the logic onto one side of a piece of paper. The same logic is shown in more traditional form in the decision tree of Figure 5.2B. Clinical trials with over 800 patients have been conducted to compare the performance of nonphysicians using the Upper-Respiratory Infection Protocol to that of physicians managing similar problems. The nonphysicians were shown to prescribe medication more conservatively and more appropriately than the physicians; moreover no patients with serious illnesses were overlooked by the nonphysicians. It has been estimated that some 75% of patients with this ailment can be handled and treated by a nonphysician without involving the time of a physician.

A protocol for low back pain has been shown to allow nonphysicians to treat over 50% of patients without the aid of a physician, while a protocol for urinary-tract infection and vaginal infection in women allows approximately 90% of patients to be evaluated completely by a nonphysician. Studies in both these cases indicate that the evaluations are accomplished with a high degree of medical safety and patient satisfaction.

Protocols for the return-visit management of patients with the chronic diseases of diabetes mellitus and hypertension have also been developed and shown to save physicians a substantial amount of time, while providing high-quality medical care.[13] Additional protocols are under development for such acute minor illnesses as headache, acute gastrointestinal disturbance, chest pain, common skin disorders, common gynecologic problems, male genitourinary diseases, and also for well-child screening and prenatal care.

The development of protocols may offer several subsidiary benefits in addition to facilitating the delegation of specified tasks and responsibilities to nonphysicians. Protocols help assure a complete and legible medical

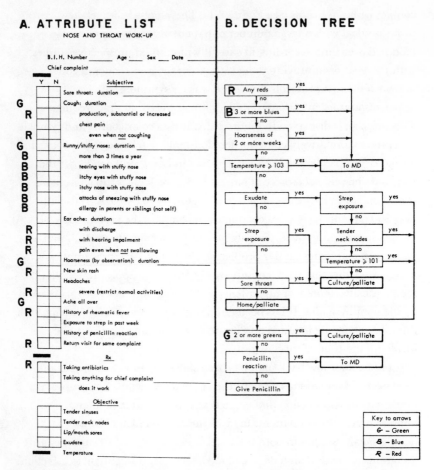

Figure 5.2 A. This sample protocol is reproduced to indicate how a "health guide" with limited training can process a patient with an upper-respiratory infection through a logical sequence of steps to diagnosis, therapy, and/or referral to a physician. B. The flow chart for the protocol demonstrates the logic of the decision sequence in arriving at appropriate steps and actions. Courtesy of Drs. Herbert Sherman and Anthony Komaroff.

record of the encounter and make it much simpler to audit performance. Another valued consequence of protocol studies is an improved knowledge and understanding of how physicians arrive at decisions and an analysis of the most cost-effective methods of management of common clinical problems. The ultimate role of such paramedical health guides, and the ultimate role of protocols, will be established in the next few years on the basis of such factors as patient response, physician acceptance, and economic, social, and legal consequences.

Similar "logic trees" have been developed by the Strang Clinic of New York City (illustrated in Figure 5.3) as an initial examination screen intended for application in preventive medicine. Such decision or logic trees represent schematized versions of the process by which physicians arrive at diagnostic conclusions. Such graphic presentations can serve as a basis for clinical evaluation by experts. If they prove effective in the hands of paramedical personnel with minimal prior training, the proposition is also immediately established that a substantial number of equally intelligent laymen could be readily trained to play the role of "physicians' assistants" for themselves or their families (see Chapter 8).

Careers in Health through Lifetime Learning

The concept of education during one-time-through schooling was tenable in the past because the rate of change in society was more leisurely than it is today. Now students often enter an educational channel at a time when there is a shortage of trained personnel and graduate when there is a serious oversupply and limited options. This disheartening experience has been encountered by physicists, teachers, sociologists, and engineers in the past few years. Conditions of living, human values, and opportunities are shifting so rapidly that there is a growing awareness of the need for repeated retooling and lifelong educational opportunities, as illustrated in Figure 5.4. Indeed, as the industrial age is supplanted by the age of service, it is anticipated that some 65–70% of the labor force will necessarily be employed in services, and many people will need to shift occupations.

At the same time a wide variety of options and mechanisms for self-renewal are becoming readily available. It would perhaps be wise to consider the initial tooling-up period as a time of "learning how to learn"; additional education or training for new employment opportunities or

A. DISEASES IN INITIAL SCREEN (STRANG CLINIC)

1 - Lymphoma
2 - Cancer of skin
3 - Cancer of orthopharnynx
4 - Cancer of larynx
5 - Cancer of thyroid
6 - Cancer of lung
7 - Cancer of breast
8 - Cancer of esophagus
9 - Cancer of stomach
10 - Cancer of colon
11 - Cancer of kidney
12 - Cancer of bladder
13 - Cancer of prostate
14 - Cancer of testis
15 - Cancer of ovary
16 - Cancer of corpus uteri
17 - Cancer of cervix
18 - Coronary artery disease
19 - Hypertension & hypertensive heart disease
20 - Congenital & rheumatic heart disease
21 - Chronic respiratory diseases
22 - Pyelonephritis
23 - Diabetes
24 - Gout
25 - Hyperthyroidism
26 - Hypothyroidism
27 - Cirrhosis
28 - Peptic ulcer
29 - Glaucoma
30 - Syphilis
31 - Tuberculosis

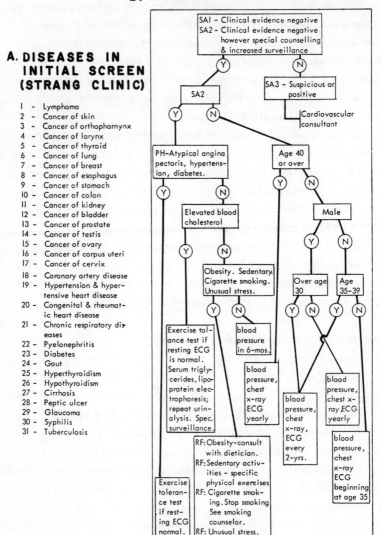

Figure 5.3 The diversity of ailments for which protocols are being explored at the Strang Clinic is indicated by the list on the left. An example of a decision tree for patients with cardiovascular disease is illustrated on the right. Courtesy of Daniel Miller, Medical Director, Strang Clinic, New York City.

broadening fields of interests might thereafter be gained through a wide variety of mechanisms in and out of educational institutions. For example, the requirements of many schools and universities are being liberalized. Adult education and extension courses are opening new and exciting opportunities. Many neighborhood public schools are being converted into adult learning centers offering a wide variety of courses. It is estimated that as many people are receiving educational experiences outside of educational institutions as are attending formal schools. Industries are expanding their involvement in educational opportunities. Correspondence schools, technical institutes, and nonmatriculating and work-study programs are being expanded. Programmed-learning textbooks provide new methods of self-teaching. The expanding worlds of cable television provide the prospect of two-way communication. Statewide and regional networks are being planned to link the libraries and storehouses of information into integrated organizations capable of completely satisfying anyone's curiosity or drive for learning with minimal exertion or effort. Cassette and video tapes will soon offer encapsulated information that can be played and reviewed at the initiative of anyone wishing to learn. Access to them will someday be simplified to the point of merely dialing a telephone number or requesting a particular topic at a library or information center. By these and yet-undeveloped methods everyone with sufficient initiative can reenter the educational process either at intervals or on a continuing basis throughout the productive period of life and on into the period of retirement. The opportunities will not be out of reach of the disabled, the handicapped, or senior citizens.

Inevitably the major growth fields of service will include education,

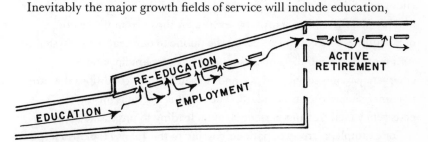

Figure 5.4 Many opportunities for engaging in lifelong education have emerged in recent years through the extension of traditional routes and the utilization of modern communications techniques. The concept of multiple careers in a single lifetime greatly expands the flexibility with which new forms of health-care personnel can be developed.

health services, information handling, communications, recreation, and cultural creativity. If the educational and economic resources of this nation can be effectively mobilized to develop service functions of value to its citizens, there could be interesting, rewarding, and remunerative employment for anyone with sufficient incentive, young or old, hardy or handicapped. Renewable education is of vital importance to the estimated 2.5 million young people leaving high school or college with no clear idea of what to do with their lives. The work force of this country is about 81 million people, of whom only about 27 million possess a marketable skill. The health-care delivery system is a major segment of our emerging service-oriented society and provides myriad career opportunities at many different levels of responsibility and competence.

The *New York Times* of February 4, 1973, contained an interesting article about 33 policemen, 3 policewomen, and 51 firemen who graduated from the Hunter College/Bellevue Hospital School of Nursing on a tuition-free program undertaken after regular daytime hours. It is significant that these "students" were "an extraordinarily mature, dedicated group with well-integrated personalities." This is a prime example of the growing trend toward lifelong educational opportunities.

Misuse of Emergency Services for Nonemergencies
The most consistent complaint about American-style health care focuses on the all-too-frequent experience of desperately worried patients who feel an urgent need for medical counsel or care and are unable to locate an appropriate source despite intensive effort.[14] In a country so richly endowed with technologies for the rapid movement of information, things, and people, there is no acceptable excuse for the current neglect of opportunities to facilitate access by the public to our health-care system. As a result large numbers of exasperated patients are flocking to emergency rooms seeking advice and reassurance for conditions that are not emergencies by any standard. The result is a serious misuse of emergency facilities and personnel, often leading to unsatisfactory care.

For example, a group of patients coming to the Johns Hopkins Hospital Emergency Room with gastrointestinal symptoms were reviewed four months later to evaluate the results using explicit criteria. The process was judged adequate for 45% of the patients, but there was no significant relationship between the adequacy of the process and any change in the functional capacity of the patient. Combining these two indicators, the researchers judged the quality of care to be acceptable for only 25% of the patients.[15] The median time spent in the emergency room was $5\frac{1}{2}$ *hours.* Since there is more than average possibility that abdominal symptoms might reflect an emergency, there is little reason to assume that patients resignedly seeking help for other kinds of symptoms would be handled more effectively in this or other emergency rooms.

To cap this overall problem, *true* emergencies are currently handled with a callous disregard for readily available techniques and technologies of communications and transportation that could not only preserve life itself but also sustain its quality.

Improved Distribution of Health Personnel

The principal deficiencies of American health care do not result so much from insufficient numbers of health personnel and facilities as from inappropriate utilization and maldistribution. Apparent shortages of physicians and other health professionals can be greatly alleviated by training and properly utilizing a variety of supplements and substitutes in the form of paramedical personnel, as indicated above. The problems of maldistribution involve both geographical and socioeconomic factors, and their solutions demand an individual consideration of these factors. The urbanization of America has led to a concentration of both people and power in the major metropolitan areas. However, the number of people living outside metropolitan centers is still about equal to that of city dwellers. Their health problems deserve much more attention than they receive.

Geographical Maldistribution of Health Care

As a result of the agricultural revolution a mass migration from farms and small towns to the cities has congested our metropolitan areas, leaving large areas of the contiguous states and Alaska very sparsely populated. This process is dramatically portrayed in Figure 5.5 by rings with 90-mile radius around each urban center. These rings, called *daily urban centers* by Doxiadis,[16] represent areas within which people travel and commute daily

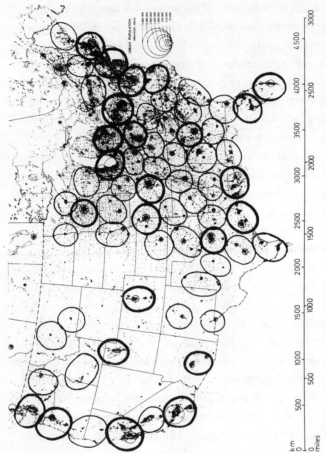

Figure 5.5 Population in the United States is concentrated in urban centers, defined here by circles of 90 miles which constitute *daily urban centers*. The thickness of the circle indicates the size of the population. Each individual dot represents 500 people in rural and remote areas. The large, sparsely populated areas are seriously deficient in mechanisms for health-care delivery. Prepared by Geography Division, Bureau of the Census; subject data from the 1960 Census.

in the course of normal business activities. The width of each ring indicates the relative magnitude of the population contained therein. Each dot scattered about the map represents 500 people. The intense concentration of people in urban centers of the Northeast, the Midwest, and the West Coast are clearly indicated. Broad stretches of territory contain sparse population and no large urban centers. They can be characterized as either rural agricultural areas or remote locations, and they are all characterized by serious health-care deficiencies.

In agricultural areas mechanization has prompted the consolidation of small farms into large landholdings frequently employing itinerant or migrant workers. Small farmers have difficulty competing and are commonly poor or marginal. The sympathy of the country has been so intently directed at the plight of racial minorities and disadvantaged people in urban ghettos that the rural poor are often ignored. For example, it is rarely noted that there is more substandard housing in our rural areas than in all our central cities combined. The standards of health and living among poor farmers and migrant workers are appalling. They suffer from both inability to pay for, and lack of access to, adequate medical-care personnel and facilities. Indeed the population of health personnel and facilities tends to correspond to the density of both population and wealth, being highly concentrated within and immediately around urban centers (Figure 5.6). The surplus of both

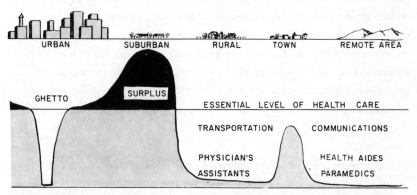

067   **Figure 5.6** The maldistribution of health personnel and facilities results from surpluses in or
068   near cities and deficiencies outside them. Paramedical personnel, communications networks,
069   and transportation are the principal mechanisms for filling in the large gaps between what is
070   available and what is needed for health care in remote and rural areas.

physicians and facilities in these areas constitutes a problem which currently defies solution.

Some smaller towns contain adequate medical care, but in many parts of the Midwest and Southwest, and in the Rocky Mountain area, thousands of counties have no physician at all. Many of the more prosperous communities in these areas have unsuccessfully attempted to attract physicians by building hospitals or clinics and guaranteeing income. There are various reasons for the failure of such incentives: Rural physicians are often solely responsible for large populations spread over vast areas, so they tend to be overburdened and under unremitting pressure. Their remuneration is small compared with that of their urban colleagues, and they must function without the convenience and support of modern hospitals and sophisticated health facilities and services. They deal with a very large number of routine, mundane, and even trivial problems that are neither intellectually stimulating nor professionally satisfying. Isolated from medical centers, they quickly fall behind the rapid surges of scientific progress. They have difficulty finding substitutes to allow for vacations or periods of study and rarely have time to enjoy the financial fruits of their efforts. It is no wonder that free choice so commonly favors suburban practice.

A variety of experimental prototypes are being explored in an attempt to encourage health professionals to choose rural or remote areas after graduation. In the Medex program, for example, physicians' assistants are chosen from among highly experienced medical corpsmen after their discharge from the military. After intense coursework in medical centers they complete their training by working with rural physicians who have agreed to employ them for at least a minimal period. These men have demonstrated an ability to assume a great deal of responsibility and have received enthusiastic acceptance from both physicians and patients.[10]

Remote areas
In many regions of the United States people live in such geographic isolation that transportation becomes a serious impediment to adequate health care. Two examples will illustrate some of the approaches that are currently being investigated in efforts to alleviate this problem.

About 10,000 Papagos Indians living on a large reservation in New

Mexico are now covered by a comprehensive, computerized health-care and information program in an experimental prototype devised by the Bureau of Indian Affairs.[17] Comprehensive health records are fed into terminals on the reservation and stored in a computer center in Tucson. Past and current patient data can be retrieved as needed from this system, which would be impressive even in a metropolitan medical center.

The problems of providing adequate health care in Alaska are monumental. In many remote villages the principal means of contact with the outside world is through radio communication. People designated as health aides have proven their value here, obtaining guidance from medical installations and following instructions in the management of the various kinds of problems—severe and simple—encountered in undeveloped areas. Unfortunately radio communication is frequently interrupted, often for days at a time, by the electrical interference accompanying the aurora borealis. To improve communications reliability a "stationary" satellite, positioned over Alaska, is being time-shared to accommodate the needs of the more remote villages (see below).

These successful prototypes, utilizing a computer in Tucson and a satellite in Alaska, should provide experience that will eventually lead to improved health care in all rural areas of the United States.

Communications networks

During most of his history human communication has been limited by the range of man's voice or the speed of his travel (Figure 5.7). Transportation of people or things was rarely faster than fifteen miles an hour until the last century or so. During the memory of men alive today worldwide telecommunications networks have been developed that can convey words and pictures almost instantaneously to all parts of the globe. Deep-space probes have sent back information from the planets, and signals from the outer limits of space are now regularly received. It is a tragedy that such enormous strides in both communications and transportation capabilities have not yet been effectively utilized for health-care delivery mechanisms. Thousands of patients are jeopardized daily by the lack of the simplest radio communications. At long last the government is providing financial incentives for hospitals and ambulances to purchase radios, but without a comprehensive policy or plan to avoid fragmentation and serious

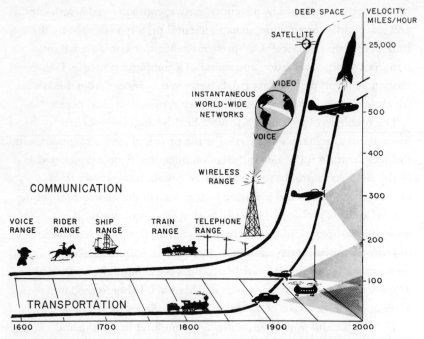

Figure 5.7 Rapid progress in both communications and transportation techniques during the past fifty years has made it possible to transmit words and pictures worldwide almost instantaneously. Transportation of both people and things can occur very rapidly over very large distances. Unfortunately these advanced technologies have not been applied effectively to improving the distribution of health care in rural and remote areas, central cities, or on the nation's highways. Data from John McHale, *World Facts and Trends* (New York: Macmillan, 1972).

incompatibility. Current efforts are inadequate to meet the need for carefully planned communication networks that fully cover the individual "daily urban areas" illustrated in Figure 5.5. These should be interlinked to take full advantage of regional facilities for the good of all the inhabitants. In addition readily available communications and transportation mechanisms can make it possible for many patients to be safely managed at home, thereby avoiding huge hospital costs.

In one important experiment the most powerful NASA communications satellite (ATS-F) has been placed in orbit 22,300 miles above the equator to serve 23 different users in Appalachia, the Rocky Mountains, and Alaska with two-way color broadcasts. This satellite will permit direct communication between faculty and students at the University of Alaska in Fairbanks and faculty at the University of Washington in Seattle. On other scheduled days direct communication will be established with students and physicians at the Family Medicine Clinic in remote Omak, Washington, to test the feasibility of teaching and consultation by satellite.

Telecommunications can also be of value in avoiding some of the professional isolation experienced by rural physicians. For example, the University of Alabama Medical School has established a program called MIST (Medical Information Service via Telephone) by which a WATS line is open 24 hours a day every day from any part of the state. An operator receives calls from physicians and refers them to appropriate members of the medical school staff using an electronic paging system. In the first year there were 20 calls a day; now there are 350 calls a day. Over a 19-month period 4,000 calls were received from approximately one-third of all the physicians in Alabama. Most inquiries involve specific questions about patients at hand. Under such conditions patients can derive some of the benefits of traveling to a medical center without moving out of a chair.

Telecommunications lines are also being utilized to convey patient data directly from coronary-care units in small hospitals to computer analyzing systems in more distant, larger hospitals. Experimental applications of picturephones are being explored at the Billings Hospital in Chicago, where x-ray images are transmitted from the emergency ward directly to the desk of a radiologist in another part of the hospital.

The transmission of pictorial, graphic, and numerical data from isolated places to medical centers constitutes the best hope of providing reasonable access to good medical care in many rural and remote areas of the world. The requirements for effective utilization of telecommunications warrants comprehensive and intensive study to take maximal advantage of the rapid development they will undergo in the next decade or so. For example, the information-carrying capacity of the telephone system in this country is enormous now, but it is projected to *triple* by the mid-1980s. If medical requirements can be specified and appropriate resources mobilized at both federal and local levels, full advantage of this enormous expansion could greatly reduce the cost and improve the effectiveness of health-care delivery nationwide. As one example, a new type of cable (L-5) consisting of a hollow copper-lined pipe is under development that will handle 90,000 messages simultaneously using high-frequency radio waves. Three domestic satellites similar to that positioned over Alaska are planned to orbit at fixed positions 26,000 miles up to serve as relay stations. Given such developments, we can anticipate that an increasingly important role will be played by paramedical personnel employing standardized and easily communicable protocols such as those illustrated in Figures 5.2 and 5.3.

Communication between health-care facilities is of extremely great importance, but additional opportunities to upgrade information management *within* these institutions are of equal importance. The current laborious practice of recording information by hand in voluminous bulky charts is costly, replete with errors, and sadly inefficient for either information storage or retrieval. Modern information-handling technologies are being intensively explored in many institutions.

Transportation capabilities

The velocity of human travel has increased during recent decades from the "breathtaking speed" of 15–25 miles per hour of early locomotives to the speeds achieved in automobiles, aircraft, and rockets. The sick and wounded can now be transported in motor vehicles at a speed of 70–100 mph for short distances and at jet-aircraft speed (550–650 mph) over longer stretches. For the most common needs private cars, ambulances, and emergency vehicles are sufficiently fast. Improved equipment and facilities in these vehicles greatly expand their usefulness. This has been amply demonstrated in acute coronary care and in the development of mobile surgeries such as are now used in Frankfurt, Germany.[18]

Experience with helicopters in theatres of war indicates the enormous advantage of their combination of vertical take-off and landing (VTOL) with reasonable forward speed in the rapid delivery of critically injured soldiers to hospitals.[19] Despite high maintenance costs broader provision should be made for a much more widespread availability of helicopters or vertical take-off aircraft for emergency services in both metropolitan and remote areas. All the necessary technologies are at hand.

Summary

The essential requirements for improving the quantity, quality, and distribution of health care in this country involve both an expansion of the number and diversity of health personnel and facilities and the construction of a new "interface" mechanism to assure that the necessary care is delivered at the right places and times. Viewed from the perspective of ten to fifteen years into the future, many different alternatives can be envisioned. There are justifiable doubts as to whether the number of family physicians will be sufficient, particularly in comparison with the health-care delivery systems of Western Europe and specifically Great Britain. In this country the best hope for alleviating any physician shortage is to delegate major segments of routine processes to other health professionals, namely nurses, paramedics, and technical support personnel. This approach is designed to allow the physician to apportion a far greater part of his time to those activities that require his unique training and experience.

Improved distribution of health care to rural areas, remote areas, and central cities is heavily dependent upon improved utilization of well-developed technologies, particularly those of communications and transportation, which can be effectively managed by personnel with limited training. This process can be greatly enhanced by current trends toward the development of decision trees and protocols that are carefully designed and evaluated by physicians until they have become acceptable as supplements or substitutes for physician contact.

References

1. Eleanor Chelimsky. 1972. *Health Care as a Political Issue.* Washington, D.C.: Mitre Corporation.
2. *Report of the National Advisory Commission on Health Manpower.* 1967. Vol. 1. Washington, D.C.: U.S. Government Printing Office.
3. Joan Hartigan. 1969. Trends in nursing education. *Ann. N.Y. Acad. Sci.* 166:1045–1049.
4. Charles E. Lewis and Barbara Resnik. 1967. Nurse clinics and progressive ambulatory patient care. *New Eng. J. Med.* 277:1236–1241.
5. J.P. Connelly, J.D. Stoeckle, E.S. Lepper, and R.M. Farrisey. 1967. The physician and the nurse: Their interprofessional work in office and hospital ambulatory settings. *New Eng. J. Med.* 275:765–769.
6. P.A. Ford, M.S. Seacat, and G.A. Silver. 1966. The relative roles of the public health nurse and the physician in prenatal and infant supervision. *Am. J. Public Health* 56:1097–1103.
7. H. Speert. 1968. Midwifery in retrospect. In *The Midwife in the United States. Report of a Macy Conference.* New York: Josiah Macy Foundation.
8. Can doctors' aides solve the manpower crisis? 1970. *Medical World News* 11:20–30.
9. *Physicians' Assistants: New Members of the Physician's Health Team.* 1970. Report of an Ad Hoc Panel of the Board of Medicine of the National Academy of Sciences.
10. Richard Smith. 1970. Medex. *J. Am. Med. Assoc.* 211:1834–1845.
11. Fred Gilbert. 1971. The use of paramedical personnel in automated testing. In *Proceedings.*

Conference on a Critical Analysis of the Cost-Effectiveness of Multiphasic Screening, eds.,
Stephen R. Yarnall and Jay S. Wakefield. Seattle: Medical Computer Services Association.
12. H. Sherman, B. Reiffen, and A.L. Komaroff. 1973. Aids to the delivery of ambulatory
medical care. *IEEE Trans. Biomed. Eng.* BME-20:165–174.
13. A.L. Komaroff, W.L. Black, M. Flatley, R.H. Knopp, N. Reiffen, and H. Sherman. 1974.
Protocols for physicians' assistants: Management of diabetes and hypertension. *New Eng. J.
Med.* 29:307–312.
14. *Roles and Resources of Federal Agencies in Support of Comprehensive Emergency and Medical Services.*
Washington, D.C.: Committee on Emergency Medical Services, National Academy of
Sciences, National Research Council.
15. Robert H. Brook, Morris H. Berg, and Philip A. Schechter. 1973. Effectiveness of
non-emergency care via an emergency room: A study of 116 patients with gastrointestinal
symptoms. *Ann. Intern. Med.* 78:333–338.
16. Constantinos A. Doxiadis. 1966–1970. *Emergence and Growth of an Urban Region: The
Developing Urban Detroit Area.* Vol. 3. Detroit: Detroit Edison Company.
17. Alfred E. Garratt. 1972. *Health Information System.* Tucson, Ariz.: Indian Health Service,
Office of Research and Development, Health Programs Systems Center.
18. Robert F. Rushmer. 1972. *Medical Engineering: Projections for Health Care Delivery.* New York:
Academic Press.
19. M.H. Weil, H. Shubin, E.C. Boycks, N. Palley, J.H. Carrington, and A. Jacobs. 1972. A
crisis in delivery of care to the critically ill and injured. *Chest* 62:616–620.

6
Meeting Health-Facilities Requirements: Prototypes and Options

Specialized personnel and complex technology for diagnosis and therapy have been centralized in hospitals. A vast majority of those requiring hospitalization for acute illness enter nonprofit voluntary hospitals. In order to attract both medical staff and patients these hospitals attempt to provide the most diverse, extensive, and sophisticated facilities and services they can possibly encompass. These concentrations of professional competence and sophisticated equipment have assumed a dominant role in the delivery of health care.

Most encounters between physicians and their patients occur either in offices or in hospitals. In a 1964 survey by the National Center for Health Statistics,[1] hospital admissions were reported to have occurred within the past year in about half of the families interviewed. In contrast the incidence of home visits was only about 2.3% in 1968–1969.[2] Despite the obvious advantages in efficiency for the physician, the preponderant utilization of offices and hospitals represents a rather restricted choice among a limited set of alternatives. A much wider selection of attractive alternatives can be identified.

Characteristics of Hospitals

The word "hospital" generally conjures up a picture of private, nonprofit facilities established to provide short-term care for rather acute illnesses. It is frequently forgotten that more than half of the 1.7 million hospital beds in this country are occupied by patients with chronic illnesses and disabilities. About 80% of the beds in long-term hospitals are occupied by the mentally ill.[3] One-tenth of the beds are operated by the federal government for its special charges (military, veterans, or public-health hospitals). Proprietary hospitals, operated for profit, are generally rare, but their number is increasing rapidly in a few metropolitan areas such as Los Angeles and suburban New York City. Proprietary owners operate 70% of the 362,000 nursing-home beds in the nation. Most patients, however, receive short-term care in voluntary (nonprofit) hospitals containing 70% of the short-term beds and admitting three-fourths of the patients for brief periods.

Anomalous Internal Organization in Hospitals

Almost all hospitals share a common characteristic which complicates administration and obstructs constructive changes: administrative responsibility and power are shared among several individuals or groups in such a way that none can act decisively to set goals or induce change. Power does not reside in any one individual, and many employees serve more than one master. The board of trustees of the hospital is commonly composed of businessmen and community leaders with authority over both the hospital administration and the medical board but with neither the background nor the technical knowledge to exercise its power. They are legally responsible for medical care, but in reality they have limited influence. Specialist groups also tend to have cohesive forces which supersede the authority of the hospital organization, and, in addition, the individual private physician retains a high degree of autonomy which can be threatened only in response to rather clear-cut negligence or mis-behavior. For these reasons the hospital may be realistically viewed as a rather loose affiliation of at least five hierarchies of power that interact for the care of patients but are not engaged in organized action toward any but the most general goals. The autonomy of the groups is so great that there exists abundant veto power, but insufficient incentives for joint action.[4]

This peculiar organization has extremely important connotations for the future. Decisions or adaptation to changing conditions cannot be expected to occur promptly or efficiently because responsibility and authority are divided. Instead issues are resolved by a process of negotiation more like diplomacy than administrative decision making. Lack of effective internal organization imposes extremely serious obstacles in the path of any move to introduce innovations or improvements in that it can be extremely unrewarding to assume initiative in such a setting.

The ultimate responsibility for the quality of care is actually shared between the medical staff and the governing board of the hospital acting on behalf of the community. This is but another example of personnel in the hospital wearing multiple hats. The legal responsibility for negligence or errors of omission and commission is similarly dispersed and obscure, contributing not only to caution in accepting innovation but also to an apparent reluctance to restrain skyrocketing costs if there is the remotest chance that an economic measure might increase the hazard to patients, even in unforeseen ways.

Causes of Overuse

At any particular moment a survey in any chosen hospital would undoubtedly reveal that a large proportion of the patients occupying beds do not really require the facilities and services provided by the institution. Depending upon criteria used, as many as half the occupants of hospital beds could be safely managed as ambulatory patients or at home. Excessive hospitalization has been directly encouraged by insurance policies that preclude payment of physician's fees unless the patient is in the hospital. Patients tend to expect or demand hospitalization if they do not feel well, especially if they do not have to pay the bill directly.

The duration of hospitalization may depend upon factors completely unrelated to the severity of the patient's illness. The physician's decisions regarding the appropriate duration of hospital stay may be unduly influenced by hospitalization coverage of insurance rather than by the cost of health care or the most effective utilization of hospital facilities. With the steeply rising cost of specialized services hospital administrators have little incentive to insist upon prompt discharge of recovered patients who require minimal care. Patients with minimal needs balance the more specialized units that commonly run at a deficit. A physician caring for patients may regard an empty hospital bed as a sign of success, but to a hospital administrator it stands as a "failure to fill." Hospitals are like airlines in that they have such a high overhead that they can avoid serious losses only by maintaining a high level of occupancy (over 70%). A substantial number of American hospitals are currently functioning with occupancy rates well below a reasonable break-even point, and this has resulted in pressures to raise prices.

The Unrestrained Proliferation of American Hospitals

The foregoing summary provides a brief glimpse into some of the peculiar characteristics of hospitals and their administration. The net effect has been a lack of initiative and few constraints on the use of hospitals as the principal sites of health care. Powerful pressures to build and expand hospitals developed as increasing costs were countered by increasing charges in a special sort of "cost-plus" economy. In addition massive federal support of hospital construction was provided over many years by the Hill-Burton Act and its amendments.

The Hill-Burton Act, providing a program of federal funding for hospital construction, was widely supported by all concerned parties at the time of its original passage in 1946. Hospital construction had been limited during the depression years of the 1930s, and a sense of national scandal accompanied the wartime discovery that 30% of the men examined for induction into the military forces were found to be unfit for duty. An implicit assumption was that the availability and utilization of hospital services is a central factor in a health status of the people, an essential national resource. At the same time it was reasoned that an increased availability of hospitals in rural areas would help alleviate local shortages of physicians by attracting some of the physicians being released from military service. As of 1971 a total of 10,748 projects had been approved for the construction of health facilities, particularly hospitals and nursing homes. This provided more than 470,000 inpatient beds. Some 30% of the grants were for outpatient and other health-care facilities. More than 3,800 communities benefited from construction funds for 6,265 public and voluntary facilities at a total cost of nearly $3 billion (with various amounts of local matching funds). More than half of all Hill-Burton projects were for hospital facilities providing general medical-surgical care.

Health Facilities in a "Typical" American City

A typical American city might have the following characteristics.[5] A city of 200,000 population with an additional 150,000 people in adjacent suburbs and rural areas might have five hospitals, numerous nursing homes, a public-health department, a state institution for the mentally ill and retarded, a Veterans Administration hospital, a military facility with a hospital nearby, and many additional health agencies and facilities. Two of the hospitals might well be owned by religious groups, another could be a city or county hospital, under new management now that "charity" patients have become relatively rare. As mentioned above, the leading hospitals compete for staff and patients with a variety of duplicated facilities including those for open-heart surgery, cardiac catheterization, coronary care, intensive radiation therapy, isotope diagnostic labs, etc. Meanwhile several groups of patients have little access to any health-care providers, primarily the rural poor and the central-city disadvantaged, many of whom are racial minorities with low incomes. The distribution of physicians tapers off sharply outside the urban areas, where 4,000 people may be served by a physician between 55 and 65 years of age (see Figure 5.6).

Although there may be five hospitals within the city, there may be twelve more small ones in the surrounding area. Many of these contain only twenty beds and some accommodate fewer than ten patients. Formal agreements, cooperation, or the regular transfer of patients are generally nonexistent between the hospitals and the medical centers, large or small, and there is essentially no effort to integrate or to share services. Unplanned and unrestrained hospital construction had produced a total bed capacity of 670,000 in short-term general hospitals by 1962, but the average daily census was only 509,000. In other words one out of four beds was empty during the year.[6]

In 1966 the Comprehensive Health Planning and Public Health Services Amendment was added to the Hill-Burton Act. Provisions were made for the establishment of State Comprehensive Planning Agencies to complement existing Hill-Burton agencies. Thus far there is little evidence that the Comprehensive Health Planning Councils have the direction or leverage needed to effect needed change. It is most significant that, while this major health-planning effort has been established at state and local levels, no guidelines or clearly defined policies have been developed by the federal government. Senator Ribicoff stated that "a 1969 Subcommittee review of Federal Health Programs in 23 separate departments and agencies found that there is no national health policy." Comprehensive health planning by established groups composed of both providers and consumers is intended to regulate the construction or expansion of hospitals and health-care facilities in the best interests of the public. Such planning is a relatively new enterprise for which mechanisms have not yet been developed.

The effectiveness of the Comprehensive Health Planning Council function was explored in one study by J. May[6] who compared four Standard Metropolitan Statistical Areas with formal planning agencies to four other similar areas without such planning provisions over an eleven-year period. The comparisons were directed toward an assessment of the number and types of hospitals, the supply of beds, the availability of services and programs, the supply of physicians, and utilization patterns and costs. The differences between the areas with planning and those without were too small to be readily interpreted with reference to bed/population ratios, services provided, the number of physicians in various categories, occupancy rates, and costs.

Thus the effectiveness of areawide planning efforts remains in doubt, suggesting that new and greatly improved mechanisms need to be developed. These should utilize the best available techniques for futures research and long-range planning. The United States is not known for long-range planning or for implementing the results of such planning, particularly in areas like health care. However, valuable lessons are available from foreign prototypes that illustrate the strengths, benefits, and costs of comprehensive long-range health planning. The most notable is in Sweden.

Regional Planning of Hospital Hierarchies:
The Swedish Prototype

Swedish hospital facilities are generally rated as superior with respect to integration, distribution, organization, long-range planning, and active research in health-care delivery mechanisms. The overall quality of health care and its universal distribution to all citizens are beyond the reach of the United States in the foreseeable future. Important lessons can be gleaned by observing their accomplishments, particularly with respect to the planning and integration of health-care facilities. In common with the British system patients enter hospitals and specialists' services through referral by their general practitioners.

Sweden is a country about the size and geographical shape of California and has a population of about 9 million, similar to that of California in

1945. Sweden is an extremely prosperous nation whose gross national product expanded 400% between 1950 and 1967. It has essentially no unemployment and a reputation for high-quality industrial goods. A larger proportion of its total taxable income is spent on health and welfare than in any other country. Sweden has been spared the ravages of world wars and supports a limited but efficient military establishment. Political and racial tensions are slight and foreign commitments limited. It is politically stable in the sense that the Social Democratic Party has been in power since 1932 with but a slight interruption during World War II. This party's candidates have been repeatedly reelected on the basis of a progressive sequence of social reforms quite generally approved by the voting public, despite the high levels of taxation required to support them. Long-range planning and strong governmental controls are an integral part of the people's lives. In such a setting it is not surprising to discover a highly organized, effective system for providing for the health and welfare of the entire population.

The present organization of hospital care is based upon concepts first set forth by a government commission in the early 1930s, whereby each county was expected to develop and support a *central* specialized hospital containing a broad spectrum of medical and surgical specialties and the most modern facilities and equipment. The central hospitals were supplemented by local district hospitals having a lesser degree of medical and surgical coverage and equipment. The district hospitals were supplemented by satellite hospitals which were in many cases staffed primarily by general practitioners.

In the early 1950s Dr. Arthur Engle became director-general of the National Board of Health in Sweden, and he has provided sound leadership in evolving the principles that are manifest in the current broad-scale organization of hospitals and health-care facilities.[7] Extensive studies of geography, population distribution, economy, and migration trends were undertaken to establish the optimal size and configuration of geographical areas for the support of health and welfare. Seven different regions were designated, as indicated in Figure 6.1A. The results of this comprehensive study were embodied in a parliamentary act of 1960. The populations in the seven regions ranged between 700,000 and 1,500,000

people, a size believed to provide the necessary financial base for an
effective health and welfare service. Each region contains at least one
regional hospital, six of which are *academic hospitals* closely affiliated with
medical schools. These hospitals are very large, generally ranging between
1,200 and 2,000 beds and have provision for all the medical and surgical
specialties, comprehensive and sophisticated laboratories, and extensive
research and service functions.

Each region also contains three to five counties each of which supports
one or more *central hospitals*. Many of the central hospitals are nearly as
large and well-equipped as the academic hospitals. Most range in size
from 800 to 1,000 beds and serve populations ranging from 250,000 to
300,000 citizens (Figure 6.1B). They also include extensive outpatient
facilities for handling large ambulatory patient loads to avoid unnecessary
hospitalization. The central hospitals contain many additional services,
including rehabilitation centers, mother and child welfare centers,
family-planning clinics, dental clinics, etc.

The local district hospitals are also called *normal hospitals*. Prior to the
regional planning these hospitals were small, badly located in sparsely
populated areas, and often lacking in provisions for round-the-clock
emergency service or adequate surgical service. They were regarded as "a
headache for the National Health Service." Many of these smaller
hospital units have been phased out or restructured so that they now serve
populations of 60,000 to 90,000 people, with provisions for only limited
specialties such as internal medicine, surgery, anesthesia, and x-ray.
Diagnostic and therapeutic problem cases that are beyond the scope of
these hospitals are routinely referred to central or regional hospitals so that
the patients may take advantage of their concentration of sophisticated
facilities and highly trained consultants.

Small rural communities are commonly served by *health centers* or
dispensaries staffed by two or three general practitioners. Health centers in
regions of population up to 40,000 inhabitants may contain as many as 16
to 20 physicians, including several specialists. In recent years there is a
growing tendency to regard the normal hospitals and district health
centers as integral parts of the central or regional hospitals to encourage
effective utilization of their facilities and a proper integration of the
professional personnel through increased communication and referral.

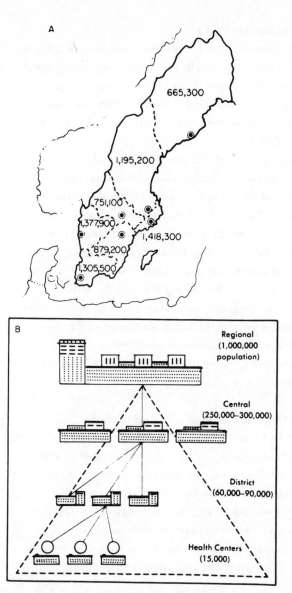

Figure 6.1 A. To provide integrated health and welfare services Sweden was divided into seven regions of approximately equal population. B. In each region one or more major medical centers were established as regional or university hospitals. Each regional hospital serves as the pinnacle of a hierarchy of smaller central and district hospitals with less complete medical-surgical services. Local health centers serving populations of about 15,000 are widely distributed over the country. Frequent and convenient referral between the institutions provides the various levels of care appropriate to the specific ailments of individual patients.

Hospital Hierarchies in Stockholm County

The pyramidal organization of hospital relationships indicated in Figure 6.1B is fully expressed in the exceptionally fine set of integrated hospital facilities serving the 1.5 million people in Stockholm County. The total system is organized around six hospitals of large size and scope, two of which are illustrated at the top of Figure 6.2. The Karolinska Hospital, the academic hospital of the Karolinska Institute, has a full spectrum of medical and surgical specialties and staff and facilities of the highest quality. Note that many of the specialties occupy individual buildings around a very large central core. The Danderyd Hospital is somewhat smaller in size but well endowed with all the necessary components for health care of the highest calibre. Each of the six major hospitals is the center of a hierarchy of smaller hospitals affording more limited service and providing the flow of patients necessary to maintain full utilization of the sophisticated facilities and services concentrated in the larger institutions. Undesirable overlap and duplication of personnel, facilities, and services are avoided by organization and integration of these six hierarchies into an effective organizational framework specifically designed to optimize the quantity, quality, and cost-effectiveness of health care for the benefit of the entire population.

Elimination of Small General Hospitals

On the basis of careful and extensive studies the National Board of Health has adopted a policy of reducing the scope of the services provided by hospitals smaller than 400 beds on the grounds that any attempt to provide a broad spectrum of medical-surgical specialties on such a scale would be economically unsound. Hospitals with less than 400 beds are thus being either phased out or integrated into the regional system as district hospitals with limited services. (Some 90% of American hospitals are smaller than 400 beds, and 60% are smaller than 100 beds.)

Long-Range Planning for Health

The Institute for Planning and Rationalization of Health and Social Welfare Services in Sweden is commonly known as SPRI. It was formed in January 1968 when it took over the functions of three previously existing groups: the Central Board for Hospital Planning (CSB); the Council for

HOSPITAL   HIERARCHIES (6) OF STOCKHOLM

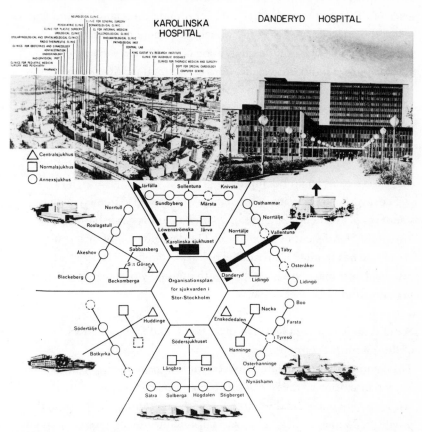

Figure 6.2 Stockholm County is served by six hierarchies of hospitals, each with its major medical center (Karolinska or Danderyd Hospital), with close organizational relationships and referral processes with nearby hospitals providing comprehensive coverage for each district.

Hospital Operations Rationalization (SJURA); and the Organizational Department of the Federation of Swedish County Councils. The primary goals of SPRI are to encourage and coordinate the planning and studies of health and welfare services in Sweden, to gather and distribute information, to help with the integration of health and welfare services, and to approve standard specifications for hospital facilities. The institute is functionally separate from the government and supports a broad program of research, evaluation, and demonstration of health services to provide guiding principles for use by the county councils and other health agencies in Sweden. Health-care services and facilities are studied extensively to determine mechanisms by which the cost/benefit ratio or cost-effectiveness could be improved.

The health-care systems of Sweden have achieved extremely high standards of excellence in terms of quality, quantity, distribution, and availability for the entire population. The development of such centers of excellence has resulted from public, political, and financial support sustained over many years, coupled with unusually effective long-range planning and implementation.

Some Relative Advantages, Disadvantages, and Consequences of the Swedish Prototype

The common division of labor in Western European medicine assigns to general practitioners the role of providing primary management, continuity, guidance, and referral, but without granting them hospital privileges. Medical and surgical specialists alone function in the hospitals. Patients generally have ready access to a general practitioner with little or no direct payment for his services. A complicating result is a steady flow of patients in such volume that doctor-patient contacts are often very short. Hurried and harried, general practitioners are forced to dispense advice, prescriptions, and referrals on the basis of minimal information. They often seem to act more as health counselors than as physicians practicing their art and utilizing their extensive training. This widespread experience supports the concept that much of the primary care can be competently carried out by paramedical personnel with appropriate levels of training.

The specialists in hospitals tend to be somewhat protected from excessive patient loads in a professional environment that is pleasant and rewarding from all points of view. Overloaded services in hospitals invariably produce waiting lists of varying lengths representing the relation between supply and demand. Patients with urgent needs are seen promptly in emergency rooms and are admitted promptly to a hospital bed if necessary. Nonemergency problems may require waiting periods of days, weeks, or even months for consultation, medical management, or elective surgery involving specialists in hospitals. Accustomed to convenient private practice, Americans would probably object or rebel at such delays. But the result is that hospitalization in Sweden is more selectively used for truly sick people, and the duration of patient stay is relatively long (some 70% longer than in American hospitals). The United States has, per capita, 40% more physicians and 60% more hospital beds than Sweden. The per capita cost of health care increased 614% in Sweden between 1950 and 1966 compared with 174% in the United States and 137% in Great Britain. Such statistics are, however, difficult to translate into terms indicating the relative value of health services in the various countries.

Gunnar Biorck,[8] a prominent Swedish physician, has presented an "insider's view of Swedish medicine" in which he offers the opinion that a national system must be based on incentives for individuals to maintain their own good health rather than on the provision of access on demand without cost. "No such organization has yet been able to live up to the expectations—and none is likely to do so. The Treasury will eventually refuse to pay the bill."

The advantages obtained by regimentation and social bureaucracy are balanced by the sacrifice of individual freedom. Critics in Sweden complain that the rigidity and conformity of their society seriously restricts freedom of choice.[9] Few aspects of life are free from public scrutiny, and individual decisions are limited by government plans and policies. The Swedish people seem to accept a higher degree of standardization and controls than would citizens of countries such as the United States who are accustomed to less governmental intervention.

Potential Organizational Mechanisms for U.S. Health Care

The spontaneous, unstructured, and unplanned development of autonomous hospitals in the United States contrasts sharply with the degree of integration, centralization, and control stemming from Swedish long-range planning. If current trends toward compulsory nationwide health insurance continue, the deficiencies of our health-care delivery mechanisms will become even more glaring. Unless the cost-effectiveness of health services is greatly improved, the country will be unable to afford the high cost of comprehensive care for all. Some of the alternative mechanisms for containing costs with minimal deterioration of quality are suggested by the Swedish prototype. The conversion of several scattered autonomous hospitals into a more compact and effective organization might be attained by means of mergers or agreements.

Hospital Mergers and Management Agreements
The administrative groups responsible for hospitals are under heavy pressures, caught between expanding demand, skyrocketing costs, and uncertain futures. The past few years have been characterized by mergers of industrial concerns in large numbers for many of the same reasons. A merger may be defined as the absorption of one corporation by another in which one only retains the name and identity. A small but expanding number of hospital mergers are being reported, and this could be a significant trend. Interest is sufficient to have stimulated the National Center for Health Services Research and Development to publish some guidelines for hospital mergers.[10] Potential advantages include improved facilities and services for the patient, better utilization of resources for the community, more comprehensive services and improved working relations for the medical staff, and improved administrative structure for internal and external interactions.

Mergers between hospitals that offer similar services to the citizens in a common geographical area provide a mechanism for reducing undesirable duplication and costly underutilization through consolidation, as illustrated schematically in Figure 6.3. Consider five hospitals in the "typical community" described above, each tending to provide roughly the same selection of medical and surgical services. This dispersion of effort inevitably produces small departments and laboratories that tend to be underutilized and inefficient. However, the development of either a merger or a mutually advantageous agreement could permit the consolidation of certain services in each hospital in accordance with their particular strengths. By this mechanism related medical or surgical

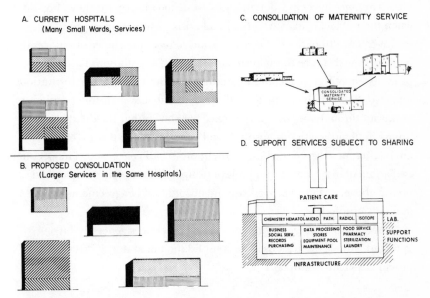

Figure 6.3 A. Most American communities are served by several hospitals with similar facilities providing similar services so that competition dominates and cooperation is the exception. B. Consolidation of services can be attained through mergers to the mutual advantage of all concerned. C. Consolidation of maternity services provides the greater efficiency and effectiveness of a larger unit and eliminates the waste and deficits characteristic of small units. D. Support services provide many opportunities for increased efficiency and lower costs through amalgamation and sharing of services.

services can be accommodated in a single hospital, thereby decreasing the number of services and increasing their size to provide more efficient and effective health-care delivery for the community. The theoretical advantages of this approach are represented by the consolidation patterns in Figure 6.3. For example, it is simple to imagine the consolidation of all the maternity and pediatrics services in one hospital, of specialized surgery in another, of orthopedics and rehabilitation in a third, and of intermediate and extended care in a fourth. It seems noteworthy that the successful merger of five hospitals, with amalgamation and concentration of their individual services into larger blocks, can begin to convert several autonomous, competitive, and inefficient hospitals into an integrated hierarchy more nearly like that in Sweden.

Difficulties and Disadvantages of Mergers or Agreements

Disadvantages develop when mergers occur too quickly (as they often do when their object is to avert a financial crisis). Mergers may produce inconvenience to patients if consolidation reduces the choice of services or increases the distance to the nearest hospital. If negotiations fail to progress smoothly, long-standing antagonisms may disrupt the institutions involved. Some of the medical staff are bound to lose preferred positions or authority through mergers. Experience has shown that the divided and fragmented authorities in hospitals will complicate the process of amalgamation despite the best of intentions by all concerned. The peculiar and anomalous organizational relationships within hospitals, described briefly above, seriously complicate the negotiation of agreements between different hospitals.

Cooperation, amalgamation, or sharing of services generally involves long and tedious discussions. The consolidation of maternity services provides a clear example.

Consolidation of Maternity Services

Small maternity services in typical American hospitals characteristically have poor occupancy rates and sustain large deficits. Studies have shown that maternity departments serving between 1,000 and 3,000 patients per year can provide better service at decidedly reduced costs. In one study John Thompson and Robert Fetter[11] divided the 33 hospitals in Connecticut into three groups according to the number of patients served per year. It was found that the cost of small maternity services (less than 1,000 patients per year) was nearly 70% higher per patient than the cost of large services (more than 2,000 patients per year). The occupancy rate can be improved and the number of delivery rooms reduced significantly by using larger maternity departments. The Hospital Planning and Review Council of Southern New York arrived at similar conclusions.[12] They recommended that it would be desirable to have no maternity units with fewer than 2,000 deliveries annually. Such units would be able to meet admission demands and still operate at 70–75% occupancy 330 days a year.

The concept of consolidating maternity services is easier to picture (Figure 6.3C) than to accomplish. However, hospitals in Michigan have been consolidating obstetric services, resulting in lower maternal mortality, improved maternal care, and reduced costs (see *Hospital Tribune*, August 13, 1973). In six years 33 obstetric departments containing 427 beds have been closed, primarily through consolidation. These efforts were strongly approved by the American College of Obstetricians and Gynecologists. One powerful stimulus stemmed from data indicating that the maternal death rate in small hospitals (with fewer than 100 births) was nearly triple that of larger hospitals with more than 2,000 annual deliveries. Extremely powerful incentives for major change are being generated by economic, social, and political pressures.

Shared Support Services

A large share of the facilities and services in hospitals correspond to production-oriented functions that are not directly involved in patient care (Figure 6.3D). Many of these functions are subject to the large scale and highly efficient techniques employed by any well-organized commercial enterprise. Important economies can be achieved if the volume of these services can be increased above the critical levels that would justify automation and improved organization. Food services, laundries, clinical laboratories, data management, and accounting can all be considered as candidates for sharing that would not jeopardize the quality of patient care. Mark Blumberg[13] elicited an astonishing array of functions that can be or have been shared by hospitals on the basis of a study supported by the Bureau of State Services (PHS) in 1963–1964 (see Table 6.1). Few such consolidations have been tried out in large-scale programs in the United States, but foreign hospitals offer interesting prototypes.

Foreign Prototypes of Shared Services

A variety of successful experiments in centralizing hospital services may be found in Europe. Laundry and laboratory services at one hospital may be expanded to cover several other adjacent units and increase the total number of beds being served. Scotland and England have a national health service and a variety of schemes for sharing services. In the British Isles a central frozen-meal system has been developed at Darence Park Hospital that is capable of utilizing a single continuous cooker for both boiling and frying, preserving foods by means of fast freezing. With a

Table 6.1
Activities Susceptible to Sharing by Several Hospitals

Hospital Administration
1. Combined administration
2. Industrial engineering efforts
3. Legal services
4. Public relations
5. Legislative representation
6. Accreditation
7. Liability insurance

Business Services
1. Data-processing computer
2. Payroll preparation
3. Patient billing
4. Collection services
5. Accounting
6. Negotiating charges with third parties

Medical Staff
1. Shared medical staff
   a. Medical director
   b. Chief of clinical service
   c. Pathologist
   d. Radiologist
   e. Others
2. Concurrent staff meetings
3. Postgraduate education

Nursing Services
1. Administration
2. Pool of temporary employees
3. Service manuals, procedures
4. Evaluation of procedures
5. Student nurse education
6. Graduate nurse education
7. Practical nurses
8. Nurses aides
9. OR-technician training

Personnel Activities
1. Administration of personnel
2. Recruting

3. Job descriptions
4. Negotiating wages
5. Job placement
6. Insurance coverage
7. Health career planning

Regional Planning
1. Developing planning agencies
2. Implementing regional plans
3. Designated services to specific hospitals
4. Hospital-utilization committees
5. Bed-locator services
6. Planning public transportation
7. Parking
8. Home-care services

Medical Records
1. Management of medical records
2. Design of standard forms
3. Statistical analysis

Purchasing and Storeroom
1. Group purchasing
2. Storage of supplies
3. Evaluation and testing
4. Central sterile-supply service

Food Services
1. Preparation of meals
2. Preparation of staff meals
3. Shared dietician

Other Services
1. Joint laundry operation
2. Housekeeping services
3. Plant maintenance
4. Duplicating or printing services
5. Pharmacy
6. Blood bank
7. Coordination of ambulance services
8. Laboratory services

Source: Mark Blumberg.[13]

high volume of production it is possible to maintain a continuous operation that does not exhibit the peaks so common and inefficient in smaller operating units. Central sterile-supply services are also susceptible to operation on a shared basis. C. Weymes[14] has developed a concept for the consolidation of sterile-supply services throughout Scotland into a single system.

A description of the concept of various industrial zones has been presented to the assistant secretary for planning to the Oxford Regional Hospital Board in England.[15] The basic concept is to separate nonclinical and supporting services from patient care, with a grouping of these nonmedical services at industrial sites. Evidence available thus far would indicate that such services are far more economical, particularly since they can greatly increase the total number of beds being served. It is generally conceded that the efficient, automatic, and mass production of laundry and central services can be attained in support of hospitals totaling 5,000 to 20,000 beds. By joint use of transportation systems, mechanical equipment, and maintenance personnel, then, the major advantages of industrialization can be achieved without any deterioration in the quality of care and with a marked improvement in overall efficiency and cost/benefit relations.

Organizations with Incentives for Economy

Hospital Consolidation through Private Ownership

Proprietary hospitals are playing a growing role in American medical care.[16] The Extendi-Care Company, for example, operates nearly 300 hospitals in this country (compared with fewer than 100 only two years ago). There are more than 700 other private hospitals that are run for profit. This trend has become quite controversial. The reaction to it is based on an assumption that the profit motive will tend to cut down the quality of health care when it reduces the cost. As a specific counter-example, though, St. Joseph's Infirmary in Louisville, which was purchased by Extendi-Care, attained an increase in efficiency according to corporate reports. The administrative costs per patient were reduced from $12 per day to about $7.50 per day. Many employees had been regularly staying on after a normal work day and punching out late. It was therefore required that supervisors approve all overtime in advance, and the extra costs for overtime were promptly cut in half. The length of the typical hospital stay was reduced. This is regarded as an advantage since the heaviest use of laboratories and diagnostic services that have a relatively high profit margin tend to occur during the first few days of the hospitalization. A shorter hospital stay is also regarded as advantageous to the patient since it saves him money without impairing his cure.

The proponents of the system insist that quality has not been reduced since over half of a hospital's costs are attributable to hotel, housekeeping, and administrative services where much cost-cutting can be done without influencing the patient's recovery. The average stay in private hospitals is 6.8 days, compared to the 8.2 days reported in voluntary hospitals. Finally, chains of profit-making hospitals can cut the cost of supplies through large-volume purchases. The company has saved as much as 30 to 50% on purchases of x-ray machines, operating tables, and other major equipment. The goals of bulk purchasing and shared equipment and facilities are much more easily attained by profit-making hospitals than they could ever be by nonprofit hospitals which must deal with a variety of internal hierarchies. The initial enthusiasm that greeted these profit-making companies in financial circles has, however, been tempered with conservatism as the limits of savings have been quite rapidly reached.

It seems clear that profit-making corporations can provide hospital services with savings of substantial magnitude. Controversy revolves around the question of the potentially reduced quality of health care. Unfortunately the criteria for evaluating health care are so intangible that such questions really cannot be resolved. At a time when all reasonable options should be critically explored as potential contributors to resolving the health-care crises, the experience gained in privately owned hospitals warrants close scrutiny. It is too early to determine with confidence whether or not the cost benefits of such hospitals can stand critical evaluation, but the option must be considered.

Prepaid Group Health Plans
A great deal of interest has recently been directed toward the tangible success of organizations such as the Kaiser-Permanente Medical Care Program and the Group Health Cooperative of Puget Sound, as well as

others that have been organized to provide comprehensive health care on a prepaid basis. The attractive features of these plans warrant attention and more extensive consideration. The Kaiser-Permanente Plan had its origin in California in the depression years of 1933 to 1938.[17] During World War II the health plan was expanded to care for 90,000 workers in the shipyards of the San Francisco Bay Area and the Pacific Northwest. It now covers more than 2,000,000 subscribers and is served by outpatient centers, 51 clinics, and 22 hospitals in California, Oregon, Washington, and Hawaii, with a continuous expansion into other geographical areas. The plan is completely self-sustaining. The hospitals, clinics, and staff are all organized into a *unified* system. The Kaiser Plan is basically an administrative contracting organization which itself does not provide any health-care services. The administrators of the plan have an obligation to arrange medical, hospital, and other services to meet the obligations set forth in the membership contracts. The program undertakes, not only to pay for medical and related services, but to be sure that they will be available and actually rendered. A continuing responsibility for the actual administration of health-care services is thus a prime characteristic of this type of approach. Through a prospective budgeting process the payment by memberships is a form of reimbursement of net financial requirements. Revenue substantially in excess of the actual costs, as usually defined, is provided to permit the expansion of facilities and services to include new membership and improvements in technology. The medical group is paid for their professional and ancillary health-care services on a per capita payment basis which is a negotiated and contractually agreed amount per member per month.

Since there is no element of a fee-for-service compensation, the physicians have a strong incentive to keep their members healthy. In addition an incentive formula has been worked out by which each year's revenue remains in the plan's pool. One-half of this revenue is distributed to the medical group as incentive compensation. The remainder of the pool is retained by the hospitals and the health plan as additional earnings available for facility development, debt repayment, or other program purposes. The amount of this incentive compensation varies within narrow limits and constitutes a specific incentive for efficient operation of the program. It recognizes that the individual physician influences the overall efficiency of the group and shares with the membership a desire to avoid excess expenditures and overuse of facilities. As a result of these organizational relationships substantial savings have been effected while a high quality of care has been maintained.

A California State Employee Study in 1962–63 estimated that the annual cost of health services for a family of four was $373 under the Kaiser Plan. Blue Cross–Blue Shield insurance cost $481 for comparable coverage. The greatest economy was attained by only building to meet essential needs. The Kaiser-Permanente requirement of 1.8 hospital beds per 1,000 members should be compared to the 3.7 beds per 1,000 population in California and 4.1 across the United States. One important distinction needs to be stressed, namely that a very large fraction of the membership in the comprehensive group prepaid plan consists of individuals who are salaried and joined the program in groups. The families who are members of the programs are, in general, supported by a wage earner, and the distribution of ages tends to be concentrated below 45 or 50. This is a natural consequence of the basic principles and the age of the current programs, since the number of individuals who have had continued coverage past retirement and into the senior-citizen category is relatively small. There is a large and growing interest in considering proposals that have built-in incentives for economy such as those of Kaiser-Permanente or Group Health Cooperative as prototypes for the development of more extensively distributed programs.

Health Maintenance Organizations (HMO's) and Other Options
The basic principle of Health Maintenance Organizations is a contractual arrangement with health-delivery personnel and facilities to provide comprehensive health care with a positive emphasis on preventive treatment. As in the plans mentioned above, payment would be made on a predetermined per capita basis. Comprehensive services would be provided with emphasis on the maintenance of good health so that early diagnosis and effective therapy could be encouraged. Efficiencies would be achieved through a pooling of resources by physicians and hospitals. Implicit in the concept is the surveillance of the quality of care by mechanisms revolving around peer review. Another organizational model occasionally associated with the HMO concept is the Health Insurance

Plan of Greater New York, in which the plan contracts for services with physician groups and for inpatient services with local hospitals. The prime distinction here is that the HIP incorporates neither the physicians nor the facilities into its own organization. Another option is the completely decentralized model in which local institutions and independent physicians contract to serve plan members along with their regular fee-for-service patients, as occurs in the San Joaquin Valley Foundation for Medical Care.

The various models that are being discussed as alternatives for improving health-care delivery and reducing its costs have tended to dilute and obscure the issues to some extent. If the federal government proceeds in the development of HMO's with varying degrees of centralization, a need would develop for some 1,200 to 1,700 HMO's with as many as 50 million enrollees within the next seven to ten years. To explore the potential value of this concept more than 100 HMO demonstration projects are currently being supported by the Department of Health, Education, and Welfare. Perceptive observers suggest that those programs that survive are likely to be located in affluent communities where the membership has sufficient financial stability to provide a continuing high level of financial support. This suggests that the HMO concept may be difficult to develop and sustain in poor neighborhoods or isolated regions, particularly with large concentrations of individuals dependent upon Medicare and Medicaid.

Diversification of Health-Care Facilities

The widespread reliance on general hospitals for a broad spectrum of medical and surgical services has been shown to be wasteful and inefficient. Many opportunities exist for diversifying and extending the selection of health-care facilities and mechanisms so that patients can be managed in accordance with the nature and severity of their individual ailments. Some of these options are discussed in preceding sections and are summarized in Figure 6.4. The growing importance of intensive patient care is reflected in the concentration of high technology and specialized diagnostic and therapeutic techniques in emergency-care centers, trauma centers, coronary-care units, shock units, burn centers, poison centers, or crisis clinics. These specialized facilities should be served and integrated by

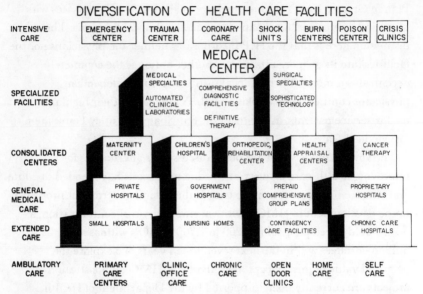

Figure 6.4 Current dependence upon stereotyped hospitals can be relieved by an extensive diversification of health-care facilities. For example, the major medical centers can remain as concentrations of highly sophisticated technologies and specially trained personnel. Centers for maternity care, pediatrics, orthopedics, rehabilitation, and other specialized functions can be created through consolidation. General medical care could be carried on by a somewhat smaller number of hospitals based on different mechanisms of financial support. Finally, extended care could be distributed through small hospitals, nursing homes, and other types of facilities.

the most modern and efficient communications and transportation systems.

The most modern scientific technologies should be concentrated in medical centers of sufficient size and scope to optimize their utilization and the cost-effectiveness of their application to a sustained flow of appropriate patients. Full utilization of many of the smaller hospitals can be accomplished by merger, amalgamation, and consolidation through the processes indicated in Figure 6.3. A specialization process could be followed to establish hospitals dedicated to children, or orthopedics, or rehabilitation, or other medical, surgical, diagnostic, or therapeutic functions.

General medical care can be delivered by a wide variety of existing or developing hospital facilities, including those that are private nonprofit, government-owned, prepaid, and proprietary. The services rendered need not encompass the whole gamut of medical, surgical, and specialized services, particularly if mechanisms are established for the referral of patients to medical centers or consolidated centers. Many of the smaller hospitals could then be restructured to provide intermediate and extended care to supplement existing nursing or retirement homes. Contingency care is another mechanism for managing patients not in immediate need of hospitalization but likely to require it at some unknown time in the future. Such patients could be either cared for at home or placed in domiciliary units (motels or housing) adjacent or near to health-care facilities. In this case there would be a need for effective communications and transportation to provide a prompt response to any sudden need for health-care personnel or services. A most important current trend is the expansion of ambulatory-care mechanisms through the utilization of primary-care centers, offices, chronic-care or open-door clinics, and home care. The many options for expanding home-based health care are considered in detail in the next chapter. Expanded self-care by patient participation and improved health education of the general public are covered in Chapter 8.

Summary

The deficiencies of fragmentation and extravagant waste embodied in American hospitals generate uncontrolled upward-spiraling costs. Stemming these skyrocketing costs will require drastic changes in priorities with accompanying organizational and financial innovations. The Swedish health service, composed of an integrated system of hospitals developed through extended long-range planning, contrasts sharply with the unorganized, fragmented, autonomous, and uncoordinated nonsystem in this country. There are many options of potential value that could help us to attain the advantages of the Swedish regional hierarchies, but any such step would require painful changes in the status and roles of our hospitals. Pressures and incentives must be developed to reduce duplication, and to encourage mergers, the sharing of support services, and the expansion of prepaid, comprehensive, group health plans, proprietary hospitals, and health maintenance organizations. Most of these alternatives are represented by functioning prototypes here and abroad that can indicate the advantages, disadvantages, and consequences of adopting them on a wide scale.

Many of these options are also mutually compatible, so that various combinations can be implemented if appropriate opportunities are presented in the future. Mentioning these various options should not be interpreted as advocacy for their adoption. The basic principle of the present approach is to identify options that appear attractive, evaluate them, and attempt to utilize those that are applicable over an extended period. .

One of the major trends of the present is a diminished dependence upon hospitals as presently constituted and a greater reliance on ambulatory care, as well as on less expensive extended-care facilities when applicable. Substantial benefits would result from successful efforts to expand the number of patients who can be safely managed in a system of home-based health care, the subject of the next chapter.

References

1. *Family Use of Medical Services.* 1964. National Center for Health Statistics, series 10, no. 55. Washington, D.C.: Health Services and Mental Health Administration, USPHS, HEW.
2. *Age Patterns in Medical Care.* 1969. National Center for Health Statistics, series 10, no. 70. Washington, D.C.: Health Services and Mental Health Administration, USPHS, HEW.
3. H.E. Klarman. 1965. *The Economics of Health.* New York: Columbia University Press.
4. H.J. Hagedorn and J.J. Dunlop. 1965. Health care delivery as a social system: Inhibitions and constraints on change. *Proc. IEEE* 57:1894–1900.
5. Robert Day, Dean, School of Public Health, University of Washington. Personal communication.
6. J. May. 1967. Health planning: Its past and its potential. In *Studies in Health Administration Perspectives*, no. A5. Chicago: Center for Health Administration, Graduate School of Business, University of Chicago, pp. 53–72.
7. Arthur Engle. 1967. The Swedish regionalized hospital system. In *Regional Hospital Planning*, eds., Malcolm Tottie and Bengt Janzon. Stockholm: Grafisk Reproduktion AB.
8. Gunnar Biorck. 1971. An insider's view of Swedish medicine. *Mod. Med.* 9:40–51.
9. B. Weintraub. 1972. Swedes discuss the impact of welfare system on freedom. *New York Times*, 12 November 1972.
10. Health Services Research Center, Chicago, Illinois. 1972. *Guidelines for Health Services R & D: Hospital Merger.* Washington, D.C.: Department of Health, Education, and Welfare (DHEW Pub. No. (HSM)72-3024).
11. John D. Thompson and Robert B. Fetter. 1963. The economics of maternity service. *Yale J. Biol. Med.* 36:91–103.
12. Hospital Review and Planning Council of Southern New York, Inc. 1966. *Guidelines and Recommendations for the Planning and Use of Obstetrical Facilities in Southern New York.*
13. Mark S. Blumberg. 1966. *Shared Services for Hospitals.* Chicago: American Hospital Association.

14. C. Weymes. 1968. *Planning a Regional Sterile Supply Service.* Glasgow: Western Regional Hospital Board.
15. R.W. Knowland. 1967. Area industrial zones. *Br. Hosp. J. Soc. Serv. Rev.* (November 1967): 2224–2228.
16. Hollis S. Ingraham. 1972. National health planning: Structure and goals. *Bull. N.Y. Acad. Med.* 48:39–57.
17. Sydney R. Garfield. 1970. The delivery of medical care. *Scientific American* 222:15–23.

7
Home-Based Health Care: Alternative Modes of Medical Management

• House calls by physicians are now a rarity, and therefore the home as a most attractive site for health care is being seriously neglected. Most patients feel more comfortable and secure in familiar surroundings. If we can identify the necessary ingredients for safe and effective home-based health care, perhaps we can find ways to make them more readily available to the benefit of all concerned. At the very least self-care at home can be improved for common mild and moderate illnesses, most of which are being handled with little professional support at present. Our health-care delivery system is not very effective in the management of the most common illnesses. For example, respiratory diseases and similar infections accounted for nearly four-fifths of the 25,155 illnesses reported by 86 families over a ten-year period in Cleveland.[1] Substantial improvement in the medical management of "colds" and "flu" must await the development of more effective preventive or therapeutic methods. The best prospect for the treatment of colds is "interferon." Current research results indicate some prospect for the development of effective and long-lasting immunization for "flu." Future success of these measures could reduce current high incidence and thus relieve both patients and health professionals of troublesome problems. The most profound therapeutic successes have been in the management of acute illnesses, particularly infections. The most difficult of the remaining problems fall into the categories of chronic ailments and degenerative diseases.

Interviews with members of 84,000 households containing 268,000 persons were conducted by trained personnel of the Center for Health Statistics, who documented 23,000 chronic conditions severe enough to limit activity.[2] A large proportion of these conditions can be treated on an ambulatory basis or by care in the home, as represented by the asterisks in Table 7.1. Many aspects of chronic care can be safely managed by nurses and paraprofessionals.

In the past the management of chronic disability has remained a responsibility of the physician, based on a fear that complications or underlying disease processes might otherwise be overlooked. (Actually this is a problem faced by the general public every day when coming to a

Table 7.1

Probability Sample of Activity Limitations due to Selected Chronic Conditions

Condition	Number in Sample Affected**
Heart conditions	3,619
Arthritis*	3,481
Back, spine*	1,769
Mental, nervous*	1,767
Hypertension*	1,369
Lower extremities, hips*	1,325
Visual impairments*	1,285
Asthma, hay fever*	1,152
Paralysis (complete or partial)*	923
Sinusitis, bronchitis*	621
Diabetes*	571
Hernia	556
Peptic ulcer*	550
Varicose veins*	535
Hearing impairment*	461
Upper-extremity impairment	401
Malignant neoplasms	260
Hemorrhoids*	243
Benign or unspecific neoplasms	227
Tuberculosis	148
Miscellaneous gastrointestinal*	958
Miscellaneous cardiovascular	758
Miscellaneous respiratory*	501
Total	22,500

* Conditions which are managed mainly on an ambulatory basis.
** The total sample encompassed 84,000 households containing 268,000 persons. Numbers are weekly averages.
Source: *Chronic Conditions Causing Activity Limitations, United States, July 1963–June 1965.* National Center for Health Statistics, series 10, no. 51. Washington, D.C.: Health Services and Mental Health Administration, USPHS, HEW.

decision as to whether or not to get medical advice for signs or symptoms that may or may not be significant.) Experience is demonstrating, however, that once chronic disease states have been accurately diagnosed and the protocol of management has been outlined, ambulatory care can be carried out very satisfactorily in nurse-managed or shared-care clinics in which teams consisting of qualified nurses, paramedics, and the patient function in close collaboration. An important aspect of this type of chronic-disease management is the education of the patient regarding the nature of his disease and the significance of therapeutic steps so that he can contribute effectively to his own health care. This process would be greatly augmented by the various kinds of health education described in

Chapter 8. Chronic-disease management on an ambulatory basis can be organized to relieve the physician of unnecessary routine involvement. Periodic access to health-appraisal facilities can protect against dormant disease processes remaining undetected.

Chronic illnesses occur most commonly among older age groups, and their management is most conveniently handled on an ambulatory basis if the patients have sufficient mobility to attend clinics. However, a substantial number of older patients with chronic illness live in institutions, and many of them have sufficient impairment of their mobility that they must use wheelchairs (see Table 7.2). The highest incidence involves diseases of the heart, followed by blood-vessel diseases, joint diseases (arthritis), musculoskeletal diseases, and metabolic diseases (diabetes).

Patient-Centered Primary Care

The traditional approaches to medical care have been widely described as *sick care* rather than *health care*. Health maintenance is a clear current

Table 7.2
Incidence of Chronic Diseases and Wheelchair Confinement among Residents of Homes for the Aged, May–June 1964

Disease or Impairment	Number	Percent Using Wheelchairs
Diabetes mellitus	44,300	27.5
Vascular lesions	188,100	30.6
Parkinson's disease	12,500	34.5
Multiple sclerosis	3,300	77.2
Diseases of the heart	156,500	21.1
Hypertension	31,100	15.6
Arteriosclerosis	43,500	23.3
Arthritis (all types)	114,600	25.7
Rheumatism	7,700	20.3
Other diseases of the musculoskeletal system	4,800	35.8
Fracture of the femur	17,200	43.3
Paralysis or palsy due to stroke	66,600	46.2
Paralysis or palsy due to other causes	26,000	36.6
Absence of major extremities	11,600	72.6
Impairment of limbs, back, or trunk	75,200	31.8

Source: *Use of Special Aids in Homes for the Aged and Chronically Ill. U.S. May–June 1964.* National Center for Health Statistics, series 12, no. 11. Health Services and Mental Health Administration, USPHS, HEW.

trend. The generalized demand for new and improved forms of personalized health care provides an opportunity for innovation too important and valuable to miss. A prime prerequisite is the provision of concern and counseling similar to that formerly provided by family physicians. Ready access to advice and guidance regarding personal, health, or social problems should be available at reasonable cost. The organizational framework should incorporate flexibility and freedom of choice so that patients can readily contact the professionals or paraprofessionals who conform most closely to their individual needs.

Humanizing Health Care

One price of medical progress has been the impersonalization of health care. The traditional family doctor is sorely missed by many people needing a confidant on health and personal matters who has an awareness of the patient as a whole human being. It seems unlikely that many qualified medical practitioners would or could spend the time required to meet the complex and multiple needs of individual patients in modern society at a reasonable cost. Experience is proving, however, that paramedical personnel can cover many of the once routine roles of the physician and that such innovation can be employed to develop close personal relationships, counseling, guidance, and an improved utilization of the rich sources of help and social service that modern society has provided. To this end it seems desirable to consider the development of *primary-care* groups, organized teams consisting of paraprofessional health workers and nurses, under the direction of physicians, to serve as an improved version of the family doctor (see Figure 7.1). The fundamental objective of such a group might be to develop mechanisms and policies that maximally humanize the process of maintaining health in terms of the physical, emotional, social, and environmental aspects of living in our kaleidoscopic world. Primary care is a natural response to the common call for the return of the family doctor.

A given primary-care group might, for example, include selected individuals with particular knowledge, experience, and competence in managing child-rearing, the special problems of women, physical handicaps, aging, chronic illness, or psychosocial stress. Mature mothers,

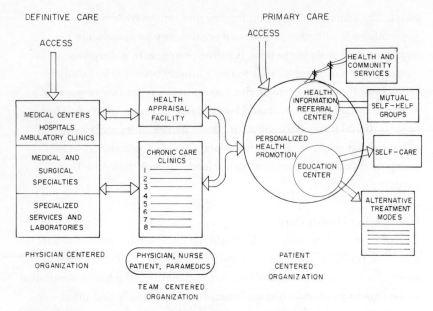

Figure 7.1 A hierarchical system of organizational relationships connecting four levels of health care (definitive care, health appraisal, chronic care, and primary care) might serve as a modern, improved version of the family physician.

the physically handicapped, senior citizens, or people who have had experience with chronic illness or psychosocial problems would seem especially suited to become members of such groups. These people would be able to bring to their health counseling a sympathy and concern that would greatly aid in the rehumanization of health care.

The specific organizational framework and the number and type of personnel at primary-care centers should be responsive to local conditions. Both the cost and duration of appointments can be adjusted to reflect the level of training of the staff so that people will be economically encouraged to use the center's resources efficiently. Regardless of these specifics, though, a large number of alternatives can be identified by which such a center can contribute to the solution of the many problems for which current mechanisms have proved ineffective. The fundamental objectives of such a primary-care center might be most clearly elicited by envisioning the role of the traditional family doctor and imagining ways to respond to the problems and questions that a patient or family would present to him. The criteria of success should include humanized health promotion superior to the best that a personal family doctor might provide in private practice. This is not an unrealistic objective.

Chronic-Care Clinics

Patients with diagnosed chronic illnesses and established therapeutic regimes do not necessarily require the direct supervision of a physician for their continued care. Experience has shown that the psychological reassurance derived from repeated appointments with a doctor may be desirable but is not really necessary. Many different institutions have experimented with chronic management modes carried out by nurses or paramedics. Medically approved monitoring and treatment protocols could serve as the basis for nurse- or paramedic-managed chronic-care clinics. One prototype tested the ability of nurses to serve in the role of physicians in a clinic dealing with hypertensive cardiovascular disease, arteriosclerotic heart disease, obesity, psychophysiological reactions, and arthritis.[3] As noted in Chapter 5, the nurses were well accepted as primary sources of chronic care. Indeed the experimental group preferred nurses as providers of many of the services formerly reserved for the physician.

A similar response has been experienced by the Straub Clinic of Honolulu, which includes chronic-care clinics for diabetes, gout, hypertension, back and neck pain, Parkinson's disease, cancer chemotherapy, family planning, allergies, anal-rectal problems, acne, and multiple diseases. Preliminary analysis suggests that nurse-managed clinics are well liked by the patient, the nurse, and the physician. Effectiveness and efficiency are clearly superior, and an overall evaluation is now being prepared.[4]

Sophisticated Home-Care Technologies

Home care is commonly envisioned as being limited to simple remedies for mild or moderate conditions. Recent experience, however, provides evidence that motivated patients and their families can be rapidly trained to manage very sophisticated technologies for life-threatening illnesses. A notable example is long-term home hemodialysis utilizing complicated artificial kidneys regularly "hooked up" to arteries and veins for several hours a day, several days a week.[5] Home hemodialysis training of three weeks' duration has proved sufficient for establishing safe routines and meticulous maintenance of the machines by the family unit at home.[6]

Hemophilia is another disease that is so expensive to treat that "self-therapy" is being explored through a form of paramedic training (*Hospital Tribune*, May 14, 1973). The necessary blood-clotting factors were delivered by mail to the homes of 45 patients, ranging in age from 4 to 55 years, for a period of one year. The result was a great reduction in the number of bleeding episodes, a decreased quantity of materials injected, and a 45% reduction in overall health costs.

Mutual Self-Help Groups

Individuals with common social, physical, and emotional problems are finding enormous support through the spontaneous development of self-help groups. Well-known examples include Alcoholics Anonymous, Mothers of the Mentally Retarded, colostomy groups, and self-help groups for the handicapped and for senior citizens. In general the initiative for forming such groups has been derived from those affected, without any participation or encouragement by members of the medical community. One important contribution that could be made by the primary-care facility would be to recognize gaps in the spectrum of mutual self-help groups and to identify those who might benefit most from the availability of such support organizations. Among patients scheduled in chronic or shared-care services, many could easily be referred to mutual self-help support groups. Sympathetic and compatible groups with common problems could also be recognized and organized by the primary-care facility. The continuation of the self-help groups could be left fully to the patients involved, but the primary-care group could provide educational support.

Home Care with Do-It-Yourself Kits

The general public suffers from an extremely high incidence of illnesses that are neither life-threatening nor likely to produce serious complications and for which the medical community has little effective therapy to offer. Specific examples include common colds, upper respiratory infections, influenza, aches and pains of the head, neck, or back, functional disorders of the gastrointestinal tract, hyperacidity, and dyspepsia. The primary-care facility could gradually develop carefully

selected patterns of remedies for some of these common ailments
supplemented by concise and authoritative information regarding both the
nature of the illness, the kind of treatment being proposed, the signs that
could signal possible complications, and the indications for prompt
consultation with the physician. Over a period of time a group of
self-contained kits could be developed for distribution from the primary-
care facility either directly to patients who come to the facility or
by messengers. This could relieve the medical profession of a very large
number of patient encounters that contribute very little to the patient's
welfare and yet utilize very large amounts of physician time at the present.

Information and Referral Centers

One attractive mechanism for communication is the establishment of
networks of Neighborhood Health Information Centers designed to
function in the manner indicated in Figure 7.2. The concept depends on a
center in each community, manned 24 hours a day by individuals whose

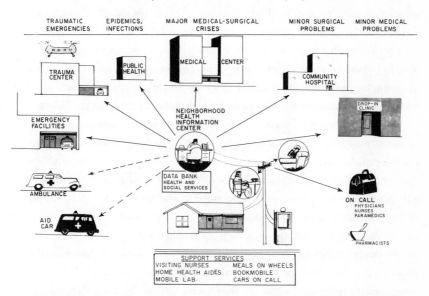

Figure 7.2 The health information and referral center is envisioned as a means of providing
prompt and effective access to the many different health services found in most communities.
Telecommunications supported by readily accessible information could greatly expedite the
referral of patients to appropriate sources of advice, guidance, diagnosis, therapy, care, and
help for a wide variety of personal problems involving health and welfare.

primary responsibility is to be as fully informed as possible regarding the immediate availability of the essential ingredients for patient care. This would include a responsibility to be continually aware of physicians, nurses, paramedics, pharmacists, and other key personnel who are available on call.

Intimate knowledge regarding the medical facilities in the neighborhood and its immediate vicinity should be known and kept up-to-date. The personnel manning the Health Information Center should have indoctrination in logic trees such as those illustrated in Figures 5.2 and 5.3 so that a logical referral can be made in response to the most common presenting symptoms. The center operator need not dispense direct advice or therapeutic suggestions, but would be in a position to bring people into contact with an appropriate source of the kind of help they need.

The staff of the center should become acquainted with people living within the neighborhood as well as with local medical and health-related personnel, services, and facilities. A citizen feeling the desire or need for advice, guidance, information, or referral would dial a well-publicized number to reach an operator on duty at all times. The operator would be able to provide a wide variety of services: In emergencies he would be able to contact an appropriate dispatcher for an ambulance, an aid car, or the fire or police department. He would be knowledgeable about the hours and location of medical facilities and about how to gain admission most effectively. He would have direct access to health professionals (physicians, nurses, paramedics, pharmacists, and others) who are on call. In addition the operator would have direct access to the very large number of social and health services provided by government and volunteer organizations in any sizeable community, such as visiting nurses, home health aides, mobile laboratories, meals on wheels, or bookmobiles.

The center could also help organize neighbors to provide cars on call for people who may need transportation to facilities unexpectedly. In most communities there are public-spirited senior citizens or handicapped individuals who have limited mobility. They could be organized to be responsive to calls from people who are not actually sick but are frightened or upset and want someone sympathetic to talk to. Such a role is reminiscent of "dial-a-shoulder" services that have been developed in some large cities. It could be a source of mutual interest and satisfaction to both parties of the conversation.

Health-Appraisal Facilities

The concept of preventive medicine has provoked much widespread interest. The possibility of periodically visiting a center where a series of tests will indicate early or incipient illness has been advanced by the development of Automated Multiphasic Health Testing Facilities.[7] Multiphasic screening continues to evoke widespread interest despite the limitations discussed in Chapter 3.

Batteries of clinical tests could be utilized more effectively by selective prescreening in which specific signs and symptoms would serve to focus attention on individuals suffering from particular kinds of illness. For example, persons who live in a polluted metropolitan environment, smoke heavily, and have a history of repeated bronchial infections would have a greatly increased incidence of obstructive respiratory disease. Spirograms have well-established clinical value in the evaluation of the chronic lung diseases that are among the most prevalent causes of disability. However, these simple tests are not commonly employed by practicing physicians, and they consequently tend to underestimate the frequency of these ailments.

Experience in pulmonary testing has indicated that among persons over 40 who walk into a multiphasic testing clinic about 30% will have an abnormal forced expiratory spirogram. More than 50% of heavy smokers over the age of 55 are reported to have evidence of obstructive pulmonary disease. Sensitive tests of lung function might therefore be set up for convenient access. A self-testing unit has already been designed with built-in instructions explaining step-by-step the process of performing the test without even the presence of a technician (Figure 7.3). Results from the unit were compared with technician-conducted tests on more than one hundred patients in a county hospital with very good correlations.[8] The concept of self-testing by patients at their own initiative might also be applied to other important clinical tests, including blood pressure, pregnancy, and urinary sugar, in much the same way that patients are expected to monitor their body weight by regular use of bathroom scales.

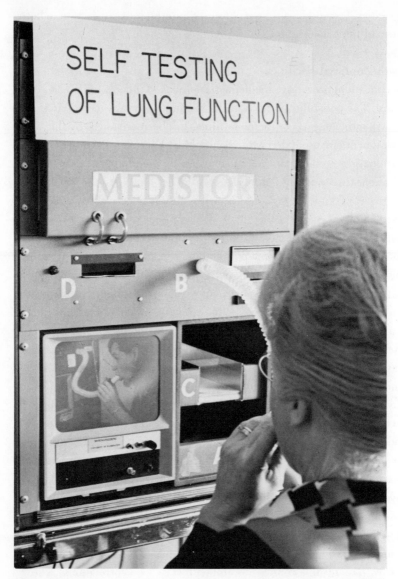

Figure 7.3 Pulmonary function can be tested by unattended patients using special equipment that provides built-in step-by-step instruction and prints out the results of three different tests of respiratory performance. This prototype was designed to explore the feasibility of periodic self-testing as a means of monitoring health status.

Improved Patient Participation Using Encapsulated Information

Our mass-communications mechanisms are capable of transmitting authoritative and valuable information in enormous quantities to the general public. In general this capability is not being effectively utilized in the area of health.

The development of audiotape and video cassettes opens an opportunity to provide frequently requested information with increased efficiency. For example, four hospitals in Madison, Wisconsin, are coupled into an information-delivery system that enables patients to receive four- or five-minute messages on subjects of common concern such as "before and after surgery," the pill, hysterectomy, and potentially frightening procedures such as myelograms and radioisotope scans.[9] Citizens in San Bernadino, California, can call a specific telephone number and request information from any one of 150 cassette tapes prepared by physicians to help patients understand symptoms or gain access into the health-care delivery system. Enormous quantities of published and verbal information have now been collected by numerous voluntary health organizations. These sources of encapsulated information in books, pamphlets, video and audiotapes could be gradually collected in primary-care centers so that patients could become more fully informed regarding the specific illnesses from which they are suffering. Referral to these sources would be one of the major obligations of members of a primary-care unit.

Alternative Treatment Modes

Organized medicine has traditionally opposed therapeutic approaches outside the confines of "scientific medicine." This attitude is designed to discourage patients from trying them even when approved medical remedies are clearly ineffectual. Recently acupuncture has attracted attention and challenged organized medical attitudes to an unprecedented degree.

Desperate patients with recurrent pain are often exposed to a high risk of improper treatment, which includes narcotic addiction and unnecessary operations. One patient was reported to have had 42 operations in an unsuccessful effort to cure persistent pain. In recent years a widespread public and professional interest has been developed in alternative modes of treatment of intractable pain and other ailments for which the standard medical remedies are only partially effective. Such interest extends from acupuncture, an ancient tradition, through hypnosis to biofeedback, a most modern addition. The medical profession is reluctant to acknowledge or support acupuncture or nontraditional methods which are not scientifically defensible at the present time. On the other hand patients flock to gain access to such techniques without medical advice, and a large fraction of them insist that they have gained some degree of relief. The common reaction that nonscientific remedies do not conform to established concepts of function and anatomy does not hold up too well since the sites and mechanisms of action of most drugs and many types of mechanical and physical therapies are not fully elucidated scientifically either. For example, the long history of aspirin began with an extract of willow bark in 1763; it is a most useful drug, but it is not without hazards and its mode and site of action are not known.[10]

One mechanism for handling pain syndromes would be to set up within primary-care facilities an educational function that would bring factual information to groups of patients regarding the pros and cons of alternative treatment modes. Proponents of selected alternatives might even be invited to present their points of view. In this case it would be possible to make the patient aware of the reservations that the medical community has about some of them, and yet not deny him the option of trying out these alternative treatment modes under medical surveillance. Educational programs could encompass electrical stimulation of peripheral nerves or dorsal columns, hypnosis, acupuncture, biofeedback, nerve injections and sections, progressive relaxation, physical therapy, transcendental meditation, etc. All of these techniques produce relief in some patients, but none of them is effective in all patients. No one can consistently predict in advance which one will provide relief. Under these conditions the medical community would be wise to provide an extremely wide spectrum of alternative remedial approaches that could be selected in controlled experiments. The results could be documented in accordance with well-designed protocols to provide cumulative experience regarding relative effectiveness of the various techniques.

To summarize, primary-care centers could provide the framework and mechanism for an extremely wide variety of essential and valuable services in support of humanized ambulatory and home-based health management and promotion. Such centers should be regarded as a multiplicity of mechanisms for developing improved and extended versions of the role formerly played by the family doctor. The services they render to neighborhoods and communities could greatly enhance and support home-based self-care, ambulatory care, chronic care, and health maintenance with minimal reliance upon hospitals or medical centers. For people with limited mobility due to either age or disability, the primary-care centers could provide invaluable support services, while additional provisions could be made for the effectively home-bound, bed-ridden, and physically handicapped.

Toward Self-Sufficiency for the Physically Handicapped

It is time to change our way of thinking about the handicapped. They have become highly visible in recent years and can no longer be ignored or dismissed as has been our shameful tendency in the past. Disabled people are extremely numerous, totaling some 18 million and representing about one in twelve Americans (this is a total population about equal to that of the state of New York). About $300 million per year is expended for their care (averaging $2,000 per patient). Despite ample drive more than half (64%) are unable to obtain full employment; their mean income is only about $3,000 per year. Handicapped people who are fully trained and competitive for positions may be denied opportunities by unnecessary physical requirements, by difficulty in obtaining insurance, and by countless obstacles of which healthy people are completely unaware. Everyday problems of wheelchair-bound people in the city include curbs, hills, steps into buildings, revolving doors, telephone booths, buses, turnstiles, and subways.

The greatest single impediment to the handicapped is lack of mobility. Public transportation is inconvenient or unavailable to many of them. At present many of these people are residents of institutions of various types, and a high percentage of them have impairments requiring the use of wheelchairs (Table 7.2). Some are justifiably rebelling against the wasting of their talents in institutions. Many are fired up by the success of other minorities in our society whose living conditions are clearly being improved by demonstrated dissatisfaction. They claim the right to be treated as "whole persons" with equal access to the goods, services, and technologies that can ease the myriad problems they face in everyday life.

Federal transportation regulations require public transportation systems to be accessible to the handicapped, but these laws are almost never enforced. In recent hearings it was estimated that as many as one-third of all Americans have some degree of difficulty utilizing public transportation, about 10% because of physical handicaps and 20% because of age and infirmity. Many of these people, denied a chance to earn their living because they cannot travel to a place of employment, must be supported by welfare. In recent years many groups of handicapped have joined together to insist upon their legal rights. They seek alternative means of transportation, consideration in architectural design, and relief from the inconvenience and the hazards of living in modern cities with their unremitting obstacle courses.

Vital Needs of the Handicapped, Home-Bound, and Bed-Ridden

The ultimate goals of health care, health maintenance, and health promotion must extend far beyond merely prolonging life. Equal attention must be directed toward optimizing the *quality of life*. This implies successful efforts extending beyond restoring function and alleviating physical and mental suffering. Long-range objectives must include planned approaches to meet the full range of human needs. The following discussion is based on the principle that an expanding array of mechanisms to provide the minimal and optimal needs of the most severely disabled would also provide support for people with lesser degrees of limitation due to age, infirmity, or transient illness that can be managed outside hospitals.

The vital functions required to support life include provisions for shelter, clothing, warmth, intake of food and water, mobility, and personal hygiene. Many labor-saving devices have become common in modern kitchens and can facilitate food preparation. The advent of frozen foods expands access to well-balanced meals, particularly with quick heating by microwave ovens. Insufficient finances represent the principal deterrent to the wider use of these options by those who need them most. Some successful prototype efforts can be cited to represent the feasibility of more effective community action.

"Meals-on-wheels" is one approach chosen by Extended Services for the Elderly in Seattle. This organization, initially subsidized by the Office of Economic Opportunity, delivered more than 10,000 meals a month to the home-bound and ended six months of operation $500 in the black. The delivery agents live in the neighborhoods they serve and become friends with their clients, who often live alone. This approach provides the assured human contact so desperately needed by most people. Such programs deserve extensive evaluation to measure the extent to which they can help, not only the elderly, but other institutionalized people who might feel and function better at home. Other facilities and mechanisms, already available within most neighborhoods, could be mobilized relatively inexpensively. Almost all sizeable elementary schools contain fully equipped cafeterias that generally provide only one meal a day. Many such schools also have buses that routinely distribute children over the school district in mid or late afternoon. It is theoretically possible that this service could be extended to provide transportation to senior citizens and mobile home-bound people to attend adult learning centers established after normal school hours and extending through the evening meal. This service could be supplemented by an "adopted grandparent" program in which responsible students are awarded the privilege of taking care of home-bound or bed-ridden patients. This valuable intergenerational contact has been neglected in recent years, and it deserves to be reestablished. These suggested approaches tend to support physiological needs, security needs, and group contacts simultaneously.

Mobility and Manipulation

The very high incidence of accidents occurring in the home indicates that there are some very hazardous areas there. Notable among them is the bathroom. Safe maneuvering into a bathtub is tricky for an athletic person and a supreme test of ingenuity for anyone with limitations in his muscular mobility. One of the most difficult procedures for nurses is to transfer a bed-ridden patient to a floor-level bathtub. Sponge baths and bedpans could win no engineering prizes. Maneuvering a wheelchair into strategic position is almost impossible in most bathrooms. The deficiencies demonstrate lack of creativity in bathroom-fixture design. One of the few studies of the human-engineering aspects of bathroom fixtures was carried out at Cornell University.[11] The requirements for the many functions carried out in bathrooms were studied, and specifications for optimizing the facilities were carefully worked out. Substantial differences were noted between existing standard models and these requirements. Even these imaginative designs would do little to solve the manifold problems of the physically handicapped. Successful efforts at alleviating the problems of patients with limited mobility in their own homes would also provide attractive options for improved plumbing for all hospitals. The rationale has never been obvious for installing standard plumbing fixtures designed for healthy people in the bathrooms of hospitals.

Holding utensils, turning faucets, dressing, personal hygiene, cooking, can all pose problems to people whose movements are restricted by paralysis, arthritis, or other impairments. Our major recreational-equipment salesrooms provide an enormous number of ingenious devices designed to make life a little more pleasant for people who love the outdoors. The contrast between this rich diversity and the limited selection of aids for the handicapped is striking.

A variety of mobility aids for the handicapped should be specifically sponsored, if necessary, by the federal government. Mechanisms designed to reduce the number of daily transfers from bed to chair to toilet and to bathtub would simplify some very basic physiological needs. Devices that can serve as various combinations of bed, wheelchair, bath, and toilet should be developed and tested. For example, a flexible shower head used in conjunction with a shaped waterproof mattress becomes a possible substitute for a bathtub. A portable toilet might be incorporated into a wheelchair. The growing demand for self-contained toilets on pleasure boats provides a market stimulus to develop such devices. We should be alert to opportunities to utilize these developments to improve the lot of handicapped citizens. For example, the Thetford Corporation of Ann Arbor, Michigan, produces a small self-contained portable toilet with Micro Rinse which provides fifty flushes on one filling of the water supply tank. A small detachable holding tank has carrying handles and empties into any permanent toilet facility. Models have been specially designed for boats, trailers, construction sites, and sickrooms.

The knowledge, personnel, resources, and technology is available to perform large and small miracles if we can only create sufficient incentives to harness and control our own organizations. These are objectives that cannot be expected to submit to simple and easy answers. However, they are proper long-range goals toward which man can direct his creative and innovative efforts.

Neglected technical requirements for ambulatory and home-based health care
People handicapped by age or physical disability have not received their share of benefits from the fantastic technological revolution that has brought affluence, convenience, and luxury to the healthy portion of the populace. Although wheelchairs are lighter and more collapsible than they once were, the basic design in common use has seen no major modification in fifty years or more.[12] It is not immediately obvious why a simple hand-powered chair should cost two or three times as much as a ten-speed bicycle or almost as much as a light motorcycle. An electric-powered wheelchair costs as much as a small compact car. The common economic excuse that the market is not sufficiently large is not clearly supported by statistics (see Table 7.2). The size of the market appears sufficient to justify the production of useful devices at much lower cost than at present. The economic reality of the situation is that handicapped people generally have low incomes and cannot afford to buy the mobility aids that would help them become financially solvent.

Mobility and manipulation controls
A NASA project has produced a sight-switch for directing wheelchairs and other equipment by monitoring the direction in which the eyes are looking.[13] A tongue switch was developed at Rancho de los Amigos for control of wheelchairs. Special patient-operated selector mechanisms have been developed by an English research foundation (P.O.S.M.) in Buckinghamshire, England, utilizing either sensitive microswitches or breath signals for controlling motorized wheelchairs, environmental controls, or typewriters. For example, four individual switches respond to light puffs, heavy puffs, light suck, and heavy suck, respectively. These signals can be used to control a wheelchair's movement. Environmental controls operate lights, bells, doors, locks. They can also activate a

typewriter having a word bank of common terms that can be elicited with just a few such coded signals. It is claimed that a good operator can type 80 words a minute. Similar projects are being undertaken by the U.S. Veterans Administration.[14]

A patient-initiated light-operated telecontrol (Pilot) was developed by Hugh Steeper, Ltd., London, to operate a typewriter with a keyboard of photosensitive cells. A six-channel system has been developed at Southwest Research Laboratories (San Antonio, Texas) for quadriplegics and multiple amputees by which breath or microswitches operate lights, radio, television, page turners, etc. The chasm between what is now possible and what is available remains extremely wide. Some of the new technologies available to expand the horizons of handicapped individuals in wheelchairs are illustrated schematically in Figure 7.4.

Security Requirements

The essential security requirements of the home-bound can be met only by the assurance that the physiological needs described above will continue to

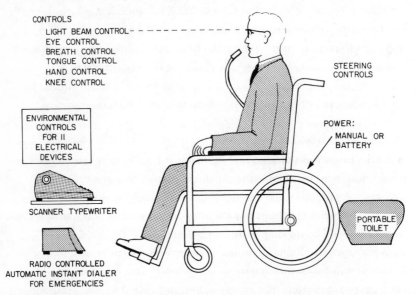

Figure 7.4 Modern technology provides an expanding array of technologies designed to improve the quality of life of the physically handicapped or paralyzed individual. A variety of control mechanisms permit increased mobility and enhanced functions, leading to potential opportunities for employment.

be met over an extended period of time. The home-bound and bed-ridden need not be isolated and alienated from the interest and action of this fabulous and frustrating world. Many devices are commercially produced and readily available to help them utilize the vast power for human contact brought about by our enormous telecommunications network.

Telecommunications: A door to the world
For the individual largely confined to bed or to his home the telephone can establish a two-way contact with the world outside. Easy access by telephone to a well-organized health information and referral center could constitute one of the most effective health-support measures imaginable for the well, the worried well, the early sick, the truly sick, and the very sick. Few people are fully aware of the many useful devices that can open this door for people with sensory deficits or muscular paralysis. Ample information can be obtained by inquiring directly to the Bell Telephone Company. Most people know that special amplifying telephones can be obtained for use by the deaf. In addition there are bone-conduction receivers for people with certain types of hearing losses. "Signalman" attachments turn a lamp on or off to indicate to the deaf that the telephone is ringing. A Code-Com set converts sound waves into visual signals or into touch signals by vibrations of a small disc. By such mechanisms the deaf know when the phone is "ringing." They also can communicate by telegraphic codes. Individuals suffering from either blindness or severe visual disturbances can still use a telephone effectively. The touch-tone system gives audible signals for each number to aid in dialing.

For physically handicapped people a variety of useful devices are available. Coordination or muscle power barely adequate to insert a card into a telephone is sufficient to dial a wide repertoire of numbers. A special dialer permits automatic access to preprogrammed numbers or even a choice of numbers. This simple attachment could provide direct access to a health information and referral center, for example. Automatic dialers (Magic Call) are available at modest cost and contain as many as 300 to 1,000 numbers on a motor operated selector. The caller need only press a button while the indicator belt passes by and stops at the number he selects. The telephone is then dialed automatically. Voice-activated telephones can be used by paralyzed patients without actually moving or touching anything.

For individuals at home who might be justifiably concerned about having a recurrence of a heart attack, a small compact electronic device called VIDA detects irregular heart beats and gives off an audible sound. The device is sufficiently portable that it can be worn easily while going about normal activities. The system can almost transmit the electrocardiogram over the telephone. Patients who are nervous and afraid of an attack during sleep could have a bedside attachment to their telephones that would aid them in dialing an appropriate source of emergency help.

Teleclass service is a system by which patients confined to hospital or home can participate in a classroom type of educational process. Teachers, usually specially trained in the instruction of home-bound students, have a console arranged so that they can communicate individually or collectively with a group of up to about twenty people. Each student can actively participate in both instruction and recitation. The teacher can divide the class into smaller groups by simple switching. He can also utilize tape-recorded presentations prepared especially for the purpose. By such means both young and old can receive the stimulation of group learning. Our current capabilities are impressive enough, but they are only a sample of even more exciting future prospects.

Social Needs
Individuals with limited mobility face special problems in their inter-personal relationships. They are not free to meet and compete with the same variety of people that are encountered by those with normal function and mobility. Our telecommunications capability provides many opportunities for individuals with limited mobility to interact with people near and at a distance.

Access to community health and social services
The telephone provides opportunities to gain access to a rich supply of organizations and agencies designed specifically to come to the aid of people with personal, physical, economic, and psychosocial problems. Traditional medical practice has not accepted responsibility for

channeling patients to appropriate service agencies and organizations.
Indeed such services have become so numerous and are so lacking in
coordination that they are usually not effectively utilized. The Seattle–
King County area, for example, contains an assortment of 1,500 health
and social-service organizations assembled in a roster in a computer
program by the Easter Seal Aid Society. No one has any clear idea of what
the individual organizations can actually offer in many instances. There is
a serious gap in our ability to direct people to those organizations that are
equipped and ready to help. A very large fraction of these services are
related to health directly or indirectly. The needs are great, the resources
are enormous, but they must be more effectively matched. This
phenomenon is not unique to any one community.

The Health and Community Services Council of Honolulu, Hawaii,
operates a centralized telephone service for individuals, professionals, or
agencies seeking information regarding community services or systems
dealing with personal problems. Two to four trained operators are on duty
at the telephones 24 hours a day. They provide a prompt response to
individuals who are undergoing emotional stress. In addition they have an
extensive file containing basic information regarding 825 different
organizations offering a very large spectrum of services, listed under 89
headings. A large number of these headings are related to physical and
mental health, as indicated in Table 7.3. The plethora of organizations
under some headings presents problems of usage. For example, a serious
dilemma is posed by the need to select the most appropriate referral for the
individual seeking counseling (71 organizations), drug-abuse information
(43), and psychiatric services (15), unless the operator has had extensive
information or experience concerning the type, quality, and character of
the services rendered by each of them.

During the year 1971 this large group of services was utilized by 2,200
professional people and 10,630 individuals seeking information (85% of
these were successfully referred or given appropriate information). If all
these referrals were distributed evenly among the 825 organizations, this
would be equivalent to less than three professional calls per year and less
than thirteen individual calls per year for each organization. It is clear
that many of the organizations must have received requests from many
indirect and informal sources. Others are undoubtedly underutilized and

Table 7.3
Services Offered by the 825 Health and Community Organizations in the Listing of the Health and Community Services Council of Honolulu, Hawaii

Functional Service Index	Number of Organizations	Functional Service Index	Number of Organizations
Abortion*	4	general	15
Adoption	7	specialized	3
Aged, services for*	30	Housing	16
Alcoholism*	29	Human/international relations	12
Alien services	7	Informal education	7
Armed services programs	16	Information services	11
Black activities	2	Legal services	17
Burial	4	Libraries	8
Camps, camping	13	Living accommodations,	
Children and youth, services	66	temporary	5
Clothing and thrift shops	7	Maternal health*	9
Communications	1	Medical and surgical services*	48
Community organizations	43	Mental health*	30
Consumer services	15	Merchant seamen	2
Convalescent*	5	Nursing services*	14
Coordination, planning,		Nutrition*	6
research	52	Pamphlets, booklets	8
Correction services, courts	17	Parole, prisons, probation	11
Counseling*	71	Police	4
Dental services*	11	Psychiatric services*	15
Disabled, services for*	3	Psychological services	17
Disaster-relief services*	11	Recreational programs	20
Drug abuse*	43	Redevelopment	4
Ecology	12	Referral	13
Educational services	62	Rehabilitation*	23
Emergency services*	18	Retardation*	16
Employment services	52	Runaway	4
Family services*	22	Safety*	7
Farming	8	School health*	1
Financial assistance	39	Sick-room supplies*	12
Financial support appeal	1	Sight services*	13
Handicapped, services for*	16	Smoking*	2
Health education*	26	Speech services*	10
Health insurance*	4	Suicide*	1
Health services*	**	Therapy*	17
Hearing services*	9	Transportation	13
Heart services*	7	Unmarried parents	17
Home services	15	Venereal disease*	2
Homosexuals	1	Veterans' services	8
Hospitals:*		Visiting, friendly	2
chronic and convalescent	12	Volunteers	12

* Medically oriented services.
** See individual listings.

limited in their effectiveness. Due to insufficient manpower, it is rarely possible to follow-up on these inquiries to determine whether the referral was appropriate and whether the end result was favorable.

Despite the obvious good intentions and dedication of all concerned in this effort, a rich source of human energy and concern is not now being effectively utilized. It could be rendered far more useful and relevant to a health-care effort by setting up a specialized health and information referral center incorporated into a health-delivery facility (see Figure 7.2). It could be the responsibility of designated members of the primary-care team to select and maintain a body of information organized specifically to utilize more fully the health and community organizations that are available. By instituting a follow-up mechanism, the team can continually upgrade and perfect the quality of this advice and referral system. Note that the only cost to the organization would be setting up the information bank, since the organizations delivering the services are already available and await the opportunity to serve the public. The very process of increased organization or utilization of these services would be a powerful stimulus to the development of integration and closer coordination of currently fragmented efforts.

Self-Fulfillment
The desire to experience satisfaction and progress in a meaningful occupation or role is shared by both intact and disabled citizens. In a highly competitive society any physical disadvantage limits one's opportunity for employment. This means that extraordinary desire and drive must be clearly exhibited by individuals with physical deterrents to performance. The development of automation, light manufacturing, computer technology, communications, and other service functions provides an increasing number of opportunities for the physically handicapped and those confined to home or bed. The competition is much more nearly even for these positions than for jobs in heavy production industry. Every encouragement and opportunity should be actively pursued to help the victims of fate or accident attain their full potential.

In this period of transition into a service-oriented society the investments of money and human resources into new and useful commercial enterprises is particularly appropriate. This approach might be based in part on identifying the useful aspects of the prospective personnel's limitations. As an example, a lack of mobility can be advantageous in a telephone-answering service.

Realization of full potential
Symbiotic teams can collectively establish enterprises and provide gainful employment. People with blindness and paralysis can form mutually supportive pairs such that each supplies a deficiency of the other. A paraplegic can serve as the eyes and a blind person can supply the mobility for such a symbiotic pair. Other combinations of people with hearing and speech defects, coordination problems, or mental retardation come to mind. An effective working relationship between the physically handicapped and the socially disadvantaged might be of mutual benefit. Team efforts are essential even in businesses run by perfectly healthy people. The common goals and incentives that govern us all could provide a sense of purpose and challenge that would be difficult to provide in other ways. Numerous scattered enterprises have proved viable as sites of employment for the handicapped (e.g., Goodwill Industries). Sample services which might serve as the basis for remunerative enterprises by individuals, symbiotic pairs, or groups of people with various forms of disability are listed in Table 7.4. Economically viable mechanisms to achieve such goals deserve both consideration and action.

Health information and referral centers appear to represent a prime

Table 7.4
Areas of Potential Employment of the Home-Bound and Handicapped

Accountancy	Editing, proof reading
Advertising	Employment agencies
Business surveys	Health information and referral centers
Child-care centers	Insurance agencies
Collection agencies	Tax-return preparation
Computer programming	Telephone-answering services
Consumer-protection agencies	Telephone polls
Counseling	Tele-teaching
Crisis centers	Translating
Design and production of aids for the handicapped	Travel agencies
	Tutoring
"Dial-a-shoulder" services	Vocational guidance
Dietician services	Wholesale drug and medical supply services
Duplication services	

prospect as a type of enterprise that might best be developed by teams comprised of individuals with various types of sensory and physical handicap. What possible pool of people might be more dedicated, sympathetic, responsive, and reliable than individuals who have personally experienced the need for medical help, advice, and guidance? Experience has shown that such activities supported by either contributions or by volunteers are continually on the ragged edge of insolvency. It would be preferable if such networks could become self-supporting, profit-making enterprises. If the service is really valuable, it should be capable of paying its own way.

Computer programming, sales promotion, accountancy, and numerous other services do not depend on muscle power. If teams were put together composed of individuals with diverse but mutually compatible disabilities, supported by the management capabilities of a retired executive and sufficient venture capital to get the group started, services or light construction operations of great worth might be developed. Demonstration programs of this sort appear worth serious consideration for federal start-up funds.

Summary

An attractive alternative to hospital care is the provision of essential services to permit more patients to be managed safely and effectively at home. One recognized requirement is the development of an improved version of the traditional family physician. A realistic look at the functions of the general practitioner discloses many of his routine functions that can be carried out by other health professionals and allied health personnel utilizing modern communications capabilities. If these resources were incorporated into a well-organized primary-care unit, humanized health care could be more effectively applied to a much larger segment of the ambulatory patient population with potential improvements of great magnitude. More effective utilization of health-care resources could be attained by establishing health information and referral services to help guide patients into and through the maze of health-care delivery services and agencies. A much greater responsibility could be placed on patients for their own care if they were supported by reliable sources of information and guidance through these and related mechanisms.

Home-bound and handicapped persons, who constitute a very large segment of the population, currently lack adequate access to the kinds of technology that would provide the mobility, social contacts, and remunerative employment that could make them financially secure and independent. Examples of the changes needed to meet the hierarchy of human needs for the home-bound and handicapped have been presented along with some specific enterprises that individuals and symbiotic groups of handicapped people could reasonably undertake. An important prospect is the trend toward recurrent educational opportunities that enable people to undertake more than one career in a lifetime. These educational opportunities can provide outlets for the ambitions of patients receiving home-based health care and also serve as a major source of health-care personnel for the future.

References

1. John Dingle, G. Badger II, and W. Jordan. 1964. *Illness in the Home: A Study of 25,000 Illnesses in a Group of Cleveland Families.* Cleveland: Press of Case-Western Reserve.

2. *Chronic Conditions Causing Activity Limitations. U.S. July 1963–June 1965.* National Center for Health Statistics, series 10, no. 51. Washington, D.C.: Health Services and Mental Health Administration, USPHS, HEW.

3. Charles E. Lewis and Barbara Resnik. 1967. Nurse clinics and progressive ambulatory patient care. *New Eng. J. Med.* 277:1236–1241.

4. Robert Nordyke. Personal communication.

5. C.R. Blagg, R.O. Kickman, J.W. Eschback, and B.H. Scribner. 1970. Home hemodialysis: Six years experience. *New Eng. J. Med.* 283:1126–1128.

6. G.W. Stinson, M.F. Clark, T.K. Sawyer, and C.R. Blagg. 1972. Home hemodialysis training in three weeks. *Trans. Am. Soc. Artif. Intern. Organs* 8:66–69.

7. Morris F. Collen. 1971. Implementation of the AMHT system. *Hospitals* 45:49–58.

8. H. Kenneth Fisher and Peter McGrath. Personal communication.

9. Marjorie H. Bartlett, Ann Johnston, and Thomas J. Meyer. 1973. Dial-access library–patient information service. *New Eng. J. Med.* 288:994–998.

10. Richard S. Farr. 1972. Aspirin: Good news, bad news. *Saturday Review*, 25 November 1972.

11. Alexander Kira. n.d. *The Bathroom: Criteria for Design.* Report no. 7, Center for Housing and Environmental Studies, Cornell University.

12. Herman L. Kamenetz. 1969. *The Wheelchair Book: Mobility for the Disabled.* Springfield, Ill.: Charles C Thomas.

13. *NASA Sight Switch.* n.d. Hayes International Corporation, Missile and Support Division, Huntsville, Alabama.

14. Ronald Lipskin. n.d. Pamphlet released by the Veterans Administration Prosthetics Center, Bioengineering Research Service, New York, New York.

8
Patient Participation: Partnerships for Health

Health is a condition for which the individual must take prime responsibility himself. This simple precept has been frequently overlooked in the transition from the self-reliance of the past to the dependent posture of the present. Most plans for health-care delivery systems being considered across the country are very much dependent upon patients who are sufficiently well motivated, educated, and advised that they know when they need care and where they can go for it. Too many of our people tacitly assume that the medical profession will take care of their health and that society will take care of their welfare. In this process we waste our largest untapped pool of health manpower, namely the patient and his family.

The American public is deluged on all sides by information transmitted through many different channels of communication, published and broadcast, much of which is accurate, sound, and useful and more of which can be detrimental to health. Sorting out the reliable and useful information from this jumble requires a level of awareness and an understanding of the fundamentals of health and disease that is far from common. Ignorance of essential health information among the "educated people" of this country is attributable to ineffectual instruction. The courses of health and hygiene in schools are not known as the most exciting in the curriculum and are not always taught by the most qualified people.

The national television networks have occasionally produced educational programs on health matters that have been factual, but these are rare, often produced for entertainment value and submerged in a froth of advertising misinformation. One television survey elicited the astonishing fact that 30% of the viewers in the sample regarded medical melodramas as prime sources of information about health. A depressingly low level of information about health was elicited in a national survey[1] and included the following:

35% of the sample did not know normal body temperature;
31% could not name even one of the seven danger signals of cancer;
53% thought eating too much sugar causes diabetes;

24% thought tetanus can be prevented by washing;

40% thought that a person with 20/20 vision is necessarily free of eye
    problems;

60% thought that syphilis can be transmitted by unclean toilet seats.

Additional examples have been elicited in other studies. In one sample
about half of a group of mothers with children under five did not know
that booster shots are needed for tetanus and smallpox.

The average child will receive more "hours of instruction" from
television by the time he enters first grade than he will later spend in
college classrooms earning a bachelor degree.[2] This enormous potential for
exciting the interest of children and conveying factual information that
can have lasting values has been largely dissipated and lost. By the teenage
years an average young person will have spent 15,000–20,000 hours before
the television set and will have been exposed to 250,000–500,000
commercials. Many of these convey the impression that there are instant
solutions to life's most pressing personal problems, often through remedies
that would not stand critical medical evaluation. Furthermore the
information about health in this exposure is heavily oriented to the often
misleading advertising of drugs. The American public spends about
$2 billion per year on over-the-counter drugs without doctors'
prescriptions—probably a larger amount of medication than that
prescribed by qualified doctors.

A national study revealed that millions of people in this country have a
conviction that in solving their health problems "anything is worth a try."
Examples included the following: 42% indicated they would not be
convinced by almost unanimous expert opinion that a hypothetical
"cancer cure" was worthless. The belief that more pep and energy result
from taking vitamins was shared by 75% of the sample. Of those
interviewed 12% reported they had arthritis, rheumatism, heart trouble,
high blood pressure, diabetes, or allergies, even though their disorders had
never been diagnosed by a physician. About 2% indicated they "did
something" every day to help with bowel movements without any medical
advice. Thirteen percent used something to "lubricate their joints." Many
people believe that advertisers are closely regulated so that they would not
dare to make false claims.

It seems utterly incredible that large segments of the population have

such serious misconceptions about such a vital subject as their health and
its management. Partly responsible must be the age-old tradition that the
physician is the unique font of knowledge on all health matters. Even
nurses are generally restricted from answering questions posed by patients.
This medical mystique was understandable in the days when the
effectiveness of medical management was largely ineffectual and based
heavily on faith and confidence in the physician. However, the time is long
past due for both health professions and societal institutions to mount a
major effort toward enlightening the public about health, disease,
disability, and their proper management. With the current transition to a
service-oriented society there should be ample manpower for the
education, counseling, information-handling, and other services required if
the necessary dedication, drive, and organizational incentives are to be
mobilized. A major objective of such an effort would be to elevate the
understanding of patients and their families to such a level that they can
actually participate to a much larger extent in the decision-making
therapeutic aspects of their management.

Patient-Oriented Health Care

Most physicians seem to share the unstated assumption that patients are
more easily managed if they are kept in an optimal state of ignorance.
This assumption is based on the observation that patients are generally
poorly informed and tend to put their faith in unreliable sources of
information. (How many doctors have had the experience of being
confronted by a patient who quotes an article from *Reader's Digest* as
contrary to his pronouncement?) Unfortunately a tendency to concentrate
rather than disperse medical knowledge has resulted from this attitude.
Similarly a preoccupation with diseases instead of people has produced a
general image of physician-centered health care and a deterioration of
doctor-patient relations. The effectiveness and efficiency of health-care
delivery could be greatly enhanced by shifting the emphasis toward
patient-centered care. This transition can occur, however, only if an
increasing proportion of the public becomes much more enlightened, to a
point where they can actively participate in individual health-care
decisions and management. An expanding array of experts agree that

many of the nation's health problems are primarily attributable to "ignorance or irresponsibility of the individual consumer or the community as a whole." [3] This refers not only to the problems presented by sui-sickness but also to the vast number of problems included in the patient sector in Figure 2.5. In addition, in a patient-centered system the management of many moderately severe and chronic diseases can be entrusted to patients, their families, or possibly paramedical personnel, particularly if unsuspected complications can be excluded by health professionals.

Preparations for the Flood

Very many individuals take care of their own health problems included in the patient sector (sui-sickness, mini-mals, and common ills). In addition large segments of the population are not receiving proper care for more serious illnesses that would normally require access to health-care personnel and facilities. These major groups are not utilizing our existing health-care system, which even now appears overloaded. Consider what will happen if and when a national health insurance plan is instituted that makes health care artificially cheap or apparently free. The universal experience in Western Europe has been a deluge of patients demanding access to the health-care system for mild or moderate illnesses, so that long waiting lists inevitably develop (see Chapter 6). This means that those who need and can benefit from the available resources are delayed or denied the service because of people whose potential benefit from the system is limited or negligible.

We are rapidly approaching the precipitous plunge into this abyss. Our main hopes for avoiding the European pattern lie in greatly improved efficiency or a rapidly expanded pool of health personnel. We must include in this pool some provision for more patient participation in health management. As we contemplate the fact that large segments of our population have serious misconceptions about health and its management and other large segments lack access to reasonable care, it becomes clear that we cannot hope to bring the highest quality of medical care to everyone. A much more reasonable goal would be to set a reasonable minimal standard of health care as a long-range goal (see Figure 2.1) and then direct our efforts to attaining this objective. As Paul Cornely[4] has asserted, "It is time for us to set forth the goal of providing certain minimum health care to every person so that the youngster in Mississippi or the Eskimo in Alaska or the Black living on Chicago's South Side will receive this minimum care." Clearly this is a reasonable long-range goal, assuming that the minimal standard is well chosen.

The Physician's Family: A Minimal Standard?

Anyone concerned with the possibility of significant illness would probably be somewhat comforted if he could be assured of: a continuously available physician whom he could consult without having to pay a fee, large discounts on prescription drugs, and ready access to first-class hospitals and clinic facilities. This idyllic condition actually exists for the members of physicians' families. Clearly the standards of medical practice that are in effect in such an advantageous environment might reasonably be regarded as a long-range *minimal standard* for the entire populace.

Lewis Thomas,[5] a highly respected specialist in internal medicine, wondered what items should be available in an ideal health-care delivery system, and he therefore considered the ways in which medical-care technology is used from day to day in the treatment of internists' families. The data has not been seriously assembled, but Thomas did find that "none of my internist friends have had a routine physical examination since military service; very few have been x-rayed except by dentists; almost all have resisted surgery; laboratory tests for anyone in the family are extremely rare. They used a lot of aspirin, but they seem to write very few prescriptions and almost never treat family fever with antibiotics. . . . These families have the same incidence of respiratory and gastrointestinal illness as everyone else, the same number of anxieties and bizarre notions, and the same number of frightening or devastating diseases." Despite the fact that all the usual limitations in the use of medical care by the general population are absent, these people use modern medicine in ways quite different from those to which the medical profession has been systematically educating the public for the last few decades.

The great secret, known to internists and learned early in marriage by internists' wives, but still hidden from the general public, is that *"most things get better by themselves. Most things, in fact, are better by morning."* The internist has at least two advantages. He regards the human organism as a very rugged mechanism and he believes that most people are extremely healthy by most any standard. He is also much more able to distinguish those actions and processes that can actually influence the course of illness from those that are just "doing something" to make the patient feel better. With his family he tends to act only when there is clear indication. The current emphasis on annual checkups, early diagnosis, anticipatory care, and comprehensive differential diagnosis (even for relatively minor ailments) has led the public to assume that everyone is in constant peril all the time. The health professions would perform an extremely valuable service if they would actively disperse the aura of mystery that envelops medicine (except for the medical spectaculars that are too highly publicized; see Chapter 4). The American public is entitled to be informed with a great deal more candor about our current state of knowledge, in terms of both effectiveness and limitations, particularly regarding that large bulk of illnesses which are relatively common and for which the patient can assume his fair share of responsibility.

Significance of Symptoms and Signs

The first and most important decision in the process of health-care delivery is made by the patient (or his parents); it is whether to wait and see what develops or to seek medical advice. Selection of the specific physician or facility is often a patient decision in the absence of a family doctor or health plan. Except for routine visits this decision is based on the patient's interpretation of the significance of the symptoms and signs that suggest the presence of illnesses or ailments. If this initial decision by the patient could be based on better understanding and judgment, an immense number of unnecessary contacts with health professionals could be avoided, and this would be to everyone's benefit. The risk of such a suggestion lies in the possibility that an unexpected complication or underlying disease state might not be recognizable to the layman. However, the probability of discovering complications is also enhanced if the public has an improved understanding of the significance of symptoms.

The most important source of information for the physician is the patient. The entire process of diagnosis and evaluation of therapy is so heavily dependent upon the statements of the patient that a physician is severely handicapped if they are not available (because of speech defects or language barriers, for example). If the patient's version of his past history of symptoms and signs is inaccurate or unreliable, the diagnosis and course of management can easily be misdirected. The argument is generally advanced that the process of interpretation of symptoms is much too complicated for the layman and requires the extensive training of a physician if it is to be performed adequately. This is probably true if applied to the very large total number of different ailments and the variability of different patients in response to the same disturbance. However, a much higher patient proficiency and understanding can be accomplished with much greater ease than is generally envisioned if this is approached as a long-range objective instead of an immediate expedient and if attention is focused on only the very most common symptoms and signs and their associated illnesses.

The Most Common Presenting Symptoms and Signs

The most common complaints leading patients to seek medical advice have been tabulated by S.T. Bain and W.B. Spaulding[6] from hospital records. The ten most common presenting symptoms and their percentage occurrence are listed in Figure 8.1. Tallying these percentages yields a sum of 70%, which is to say that these ten indicators, individually and in combination, accounted for some 70% of the admitting complaints of this sample of 4,000 patients. This observation suggests that by concentrating attention on the nature, origins, and significance of even this limited list of common complaints, the level of understanding and decision making by patients could be greatly enhanced.

If every symptom and sign represented a unique indication of a single malfunction or disease, diagnosis could be simplified to a process of one-to-one matching. Unfortunately there are many more diseases and disabilities than signs or symptoms, so there is substantial overlap. Nonetheless each symptom tends inherently to narrow down the probable sites of dysfunction and to eliminate many possibilities from serious consideration. A simplified version of this overlap between the symptoms of the 4,000 patients according to the organ system found to be affected by subsequent examination is illustrated in Figure 8.2. For example, chest pain was found to be most frequently associated with cardiovascular (33%)

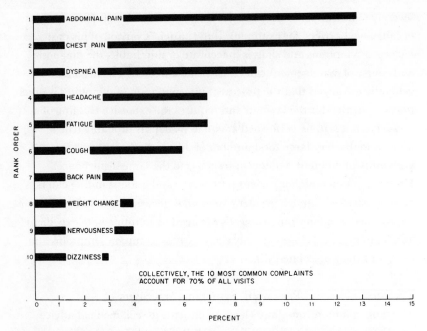

Figure 8.1 Ten specific symptoms recur with extremely high frequency among groups of unselected patients. For example, the ten common symptoms listed here accounted for 70% of 4,000 patient contacts in a study reported by S.T. Bain and W.B. Spaulding.[6]

and respiratory diseases (12%), with substantial fractions attributable to functional (psychological) or psychiatric causes (26%), musculoskeletal problems (12%), and other scattered problems (17%). Similar degrees of overlap are displayed for the other common symptoms. Of major importance is the consistent appearance of relatively large percentages in the psychiatric column, which implies that no organic cause was found. (It is an old tradition in medicine that all possible organic causes or symptoms should be excluded before a diagnosis of psychiatric or functional cause is considered.)

The Prenatal Period: "Prime Time" for Adult Health Education

Our massive communications networks could be used to much greater effect in bringing factual information to the public. This has not been tried for a very significant reason. The general public is not receptive to such information except in two circumstances: (1) young people who still have their natural curiosity; and (2) people faced with immediate problems affecting their health. If health-education efforts are concentrated on these two groups a receptive response would be more likely, and the general desire for such information could be fostered in the process.

Pregnancy, especially the first pregnancy, represents a period in the life of most women during which their interest in health matters reaches a very high peak. The current trend toward natural childbirth further enhances this period as a "prime time" for the health education of both parents, particularly in reference to such problems as congenital malformations, common childhood diseases, genetic disturbances, sensory deficiencies, and other problems of the newborn infant and young child. It has been a source of concern and shame that the United States lags behind

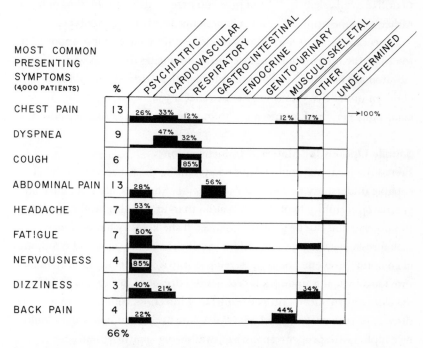

Figure 8.2 Each of the symptoms listed in Figure 8.1 may signify ailments affecting more than one organ system of the body, as indicated by the percentages under the areas of medical concern listed at the top of the figure. (Weight loss was excluded on the basis that it is more a sign than a symptom.) Despite the fact that these symptoms are not specific for either disease or organ systems, an appreciation of their potential significance on the part of the patient could greatly enhance both his ability to manage his ailments and his judgment of when to seek medical advice.

about a dozen countries of Western Europe and Scandinavia with respect to the control of death and disease among mothers and children.

Great rewards would be attained if the maximum possible number of expectant mothers could be made thoroughly aware of the major risk factors in infants and children,[7] the signs and symptoms to watch for, and the proper steps to take when indicated (e.g., clinical consultation, immunization, additional testing), and if they could be given a solid basis for judgment when acute illness or injury occurs. It is not sufficient merely to make available optimized indoctrination into health matters, however; carefully considered incentives should be developed to encourage maximal utilization of the opportunities. For example, the charges for delivery of babies in France are covered by insurance, *except* for those who have failed to utilize available programs of prenatal care. This might be considered a rather extreme approach, but it represents an existing prototype.

Expectant mothers and fathers would certainly have ample opportunity to utilize the information imparted to them during the years when their children are growing up. For example, health statistics[8] indicate that children under five years of age experience a yearly average of 3.3 acute conditions per child, a rate more than twice as high as that for adults.

Sample Options for Maternal Indoctrination
Prenatal education should be aimed at making the expectant mother a capable understudy for her child's physician. She does, after all, have far greater opportunity to observe her child than any health professional, and this observation can be greatly enhanced if she knows what evidence to look for while caring for her child. Descriptions of the signs and symptoms of common problems could be developed into a series of decision trees to provide a logical framework for sequential decisions in case the child develops gastroenteritis, upper respiratory infection, communicable disease, or convulsions. Methods of avoiding accidental poisoning should be coupled with proper responses to swallowing aspirin, disinfectants, poisonous berries, outdoor plants, or common household products such as bleaches, cleansers, insecticides, and cosmetics. Appropriate measures to combat accidental injuries should also be common knowledge among mothers. The danger to children from flammable clothing, for example, is very real.

Those mothers who would be most likely to avail themselves of health-education opportunities are the same ones most likely to have effective pediatric care for their children. A primary aim of this proposal, however, is to extend the health-education process much more widely than that. The educational program could make almost any mother's relations with her pediatrician more effective and meaningful. In addition many mothers could become much more self-sufficient and thus relieve the health-care system of unnecessary loading.

Mothers can also become more effective in the detection of other conditions of extreme importance that should be caught and treated as early as possible. For example, hypothyroidism can depress mentality, and its effects are reversible only if they are detected quickly. Some 1–3% of preschool children need glasses, but this is commonly undetected, and, as was mentioned in Chapter 4, the early detection of deafness is extremely important because it is commonly mistaken for mental retardation.

The congenital disease known as phenylketonuria was discovered because a mother noticed a peculiar odor in her child's urine and brought it to her physician's attention. He pursued this clue and discovered an enzyme deficiency that can lead to serious mental retardation if the child is not given dietary therapy. Evidence of congenital defects may be most readily recognized by alert mothers, and the recording of the family history should be a part of prenatal preparation in order to assess the possibility of genetic disturbance. The probability, significance, and alternatives should be carefully explained because important questions may require prenatal input or decisions.

Nearly 25% of all white children ages 5–14 have never seen a dentist.[1] The percentage rises precipitously for rural farm children (41%), children in the south (45%), children from low-income families (60%), and nonwhite children (63%). Dental care is neglected far more often in the United States than in other developed countries. For example, free dental care through childhood is available to all children in many West European countries. In some instances this is carried out in school health programs. In contrast dental care in this country is a matter of private concern, with the result that many health insurance companies and prepaid plans exclude dental care from their programs for adults because of the extremely high cost of overcoming years of neglect to bring oral care up to maintenance levels.

Intelligence is extremely difficult to evaluate or measure, but there is evidence suggesting that from birth to four years of age children develop some 50% of the "intelligence" they will have at age seventeen. During this same critical period the brain grows to 90% of its final volume. The importance of adequate nutrition should be more generally understood by mothers because a significant deficiency of protein in the diet during this period can have lasting consequences.

It is recognized that this process of maternal observation could cause a greatly increased number of worried mothers. They must have more ready access to counsel and guidance without an excessive encroachment on the time of health professionals through such mechanisms as the health information and referral centers described in Chapter 7.

It is not proposed that mothers be exposed to the full spectrum of ailments constituting the practice of pediatrics. Rather it is suggested that the logical steps to be taken in the most common situations be conveyed in an organized and useful manner. Serious, complex, and therapeutically challenging disease states should clearly remain the province of the highly trained physician. However, an enlightened mother with access to paramedical personnel can accommodate a very large proportion of the illnesses that beset children.

The Impressionable Years: Creating Interest in Health

The natural curiosity during childhood years appears boundless. It is an ideal time to develop appropriate interests in matters related to good health. Many invaluable opportunities are missed to attract the interest of young people to the basic functions of their bodies, the principles of good hygiene, the importance of proper nutrition, and other aspects of health and disease. Included among such opportunities are the development of educational games that could convey factual impressions at a time when children are most responsive. To children learning is still fun; neglecting such an opportunity to imbue them with sound knowledge seems a deplorable waste. Instead we provide them with simulated instruments of destruction, means of simulating adult activities, or idle distractions.

Television could be a powerful educational mechanism to bring important ideas and new concepts to young and impressionable minds. The thousands of hours a child spends staring blankly at pointless animated cartoons, stylized westerns, stupid clowns, and superficial foolishness represent a challenge to those who are looking for new means of stimulating his interest in matters of educational substance. Indeed the overexposure of children to high-pressure advertising should be the basis for a demand for "equal time" to present factual and useful information. Both commercial and public television have failed to realize their full educational potential. The newly developing cable television networks provide one more opportunity to attract the attention of various age groups to material that should be of interest and value to them. The creative imagination applied to *Sesame Street* programming should be applied to health matters.

Educational games and toys represent an almost untapped resource for exciting curiosity about living things in general and matters pertaining to health in particular. One cannot view the enormous diversity of toys and games available in any large store without acknowledging the combination of innovation and practical child psychology that has created so many intricate mechanisms and interest-provoking ideas. Consider for a moment the vast array of plastic models, working simulations of cars, planes, guns, and machines. The same degree of realism could be introduced into models of living organisms. A large number of competitive games and mechanized quizzes elicit information about science or geography or types of animals. Why not include information about the functions of living organ systems at a time when the curiosity is most easily excited and sustained? The profit motive is the driving force that can uncork this creative effort. The need is clear to develop the incentives and capital necessary to unleash creative genius and encourage the development of new enterprises, services, and inventions specifically oriented toward improving the understanding of children (and their parents) of matters pertaining to health and the common illnesses.

Attractive Alternatives for Expanded Health Education in Schools
A comprehensive program of health education extending throughout the public school career is clearly a necessary and realistic objective. The teachers of early grades are generally receptive to the addition of interesting and relevant subjects to their courses if the necessary teaching materials are available in readily usable forms. There can be little doubt

that a greatly increased emphasis on topics related to health would be adopted enthusiastically nationwide if there were a concentrated effort to provide improved teaching materials for the purpose. Appropriate texts and pamphlets, charts, models, and audiovisual aids can be used to present in clear and interesting fashion the basic structural components and underlying functional principles of various organs. For example, the functioning of the eyes, the voice, the lungs, skin, and heart might be presented through individual experiences as well as through comparative physiology utilizing lower animal forms. The sources of normal sensations and the origins and significance of certain common symptoms are not beyond the capacity of youth to understand if properly presented (see also Figure 8.3).

As a direct stimulus, the Department of Health, Education, and Welfare could mount a program to expand the availability of appropriate teaching

SIMULATED SYMPTOMS TO STIMULATE INTEREST

SPECIAL INTEREST	NEUROMUSCULAR	CARDIO - PULMONARY
A. VISION HYPERMETROPIA MYOPIA STRABISMUS COLOR BLINDNESS NIGHT BLINDNESS PUPIL RESPONSE SCOTOMA BLINDNESS B. HEARING BLOCKADE DEAFNESS FREQUENCY LOSS C. VESTIBULAR MECHANISMS NYSTAGMUS DIZZINESS ROTATORY FALLING PAST POINTING	A. POSTURAL RESPONSES STANDING SWAY STRETCH REFLEXES PATELLAR ACHILLES BRACHIAL B. SIMULATED HANDICAPS SENSORY LOSSES SPLINTS CRUTCHES WHEELCHAIR C. ISCHEMIC PARALYSIS SENSATION LOSS MUSCLE WEAKNESS CLAUDICATION TINGLING HYPERSENSITIVITY D. SOMATIC SENSATIONS HEAT — COLD PRESSURE PAIN SOMATIC PAIN VISCERAL PAIN E. FLEXION REFLEXES	A. EXERTIONAL EFFECTS PULSE RATE BLOOD PRESSURE HEART SOUNDS, MURMURS EXERTIONAL DYSPNEA POSTURAL HYPOTENSION B. RESPIRATORY FUNCTION TIDAL VOLUME VITAL CAPACITY FORCED EXPIRATION EXPIRATORY OBSTRUCTION HYPERCARBIA DYSPNEA HYPERVENTILATION SPEECH VALSALVA MANEUVER C. RESUSCITATION MOUTH TO MOUTH ARTIFICIAL RESPIRATION EXTERNAL CARDIAC MASSAGE

Figure 8.3 A very large number of interesting signs and symptoms can be easily simulated by simple laboratory procedures. If the relations of such signs and symptoms to specific illnesses are presented in a mature and interesting manner, a lasting improvement in the insight students have into their own health problems should result.

materials by subsidizing the collaborative efforts of recognized medical authorities and the commercial producers of these materials. The requirements could be based on the continuous query, "What should everyone know about normal function, signs and symptoms, disease and disability at each age and stage?" The curricular offerings at this level should be designed to provide a solid foundation for more extensive coverage in the upper grades, including laboratories on simulated symptoms and the education-for-parenthood classes described below. The fear that a generation of hypochondriacs might result from too much information could be countered by taking the positive attitude implied by the physician's approach to his own family's health described earlier in this chapter.

Current middle- and high-school courses on health and hygiene are too often unexciting, uninteresting, and unpopular. If there is any subject that should be most interesting in this egocentric world, the function and malfunction of one's own body should certainly be it. The problem might well be a persistence of the tendency to regard the medical profession as the sole source of wisdom and knowledge in health matters. As a result the material presented suffers from being so superficial as to be lacking in relevance. The background and training of the health educators in our schools is also a factor. In 1961 some 90% of health instruction in many states was given by physical educators and athletic coaches.[1] There is good reason to doubt that the educational background of athletes assures an interest and competence in conveying factual, relevant, and interesting information about health and sickness. The preparation of future adults and parents to participate intelligently and cooperatively with health professionals is so vital a function that the very best teachers and instructional aids should be mobilized for the purpose.

Since the responsibility for the management of mini-mals, common ills, and sui-sickness devolves upon the patient, there should be a conscientious effort to prepare the general public for this role. One important site at which much information should be presented dispassionately and as interestingly as possible is in the curricula of middle and high schools.

Sui-sickness should be a focus of major propaganda campaigns designed to discourage people from voluntary acts or habits that are generally recognized hazards to health. Intensive and carefully designed courses and behavior-modification techniques should be concentrated on problems of drug and alcohol abuse and excessive pill consumption. The success of driver's training indicates that this approach can be expanded to include the kinds of health hazards that people undertake in the name of sports and recreation.

Preparation for Patient Participation in Major Medical Problems

Current curricula stop far short of providing the information needed by individuals if they are to decide intelligently when to seek medical help and how to participate actively in the decisions involving, and the actual management of, those problems that fall into the medical sector of Figure 2.5. It is obvious that this degree of education cannot be attained equally by all segments of society. It is also true that those most likely to reach high levels of understanding are those who can better afford to utilize health professionals. However, the public schools offer an opportunity to present a wealth of useful and relevant information that would increase the level of health in this country without unnecessarily overloading the health-care system. Mechanisms must be sought to capture the interest and excite the curiosity of teenage students, a problem of no mean proportions. However, this objective is clearly not impossible, as the description of some possible approaches may indicate.

The Display of Common Symptoms

Many common symptoms can be reproduced or simulated by completely safe and relatively simple methods (Figure 8.3). For example, nearsighted and farsighted visual disturbances can be simulated by simple spherical lenses of different focal lengths. Astigmatism can be experienced using cylindrical lenses. Imbalance of eye muscles (strabismus) can be demonstrated by prisms. Optical illusions and afterimages are interesting experiments. "Spots before the eyes" can be produced mechanically. Pupillary reflexes in response to light can be directly observed and can be made to simulate the effects of drugs on the size of the pupil.

Common hearing defects can also be simulated. Blockage of the ear canal is easy to produce, and the effects on air conduction and bone conduction are obvious and interesting. A change of pressure in the middle ear is a common experience of great importance in middle-ear infections and in clearing the ears during changes in altitude. The effects of hearing losses can be simulated by simple electronic filters that can show how voices sound when high tones are lost. This is a subject of great importance to teenagers, who are currently damaging their hearing by exposure to extremely loud music (a special form of sui-sickness).

The inner ear also contains position-sensing organs that are of extreme importance in maintaining posture. The dizziness that occurs with rotary motion is associated with rhythmic motion of the eyes (nystagmus), which can also be stimulated by warm water or oil in the ear canal. The role of these reflexes in motion sickness (and hangovers) should be of interest to teenagers. The effects of alcohol on coordination or on the functions needed for safe driving might be demonstrated as an object lesson. Factual information about the effects of various common and dangerous drugs might be included in such presentations as an incentive to avoid sui-sickness from such agents.

Postural reflexes in the extremities can be easily reproduced by tapping appropriate tendons. In addition the problems presented by physical handicaps can be simulated by having normal individuals wear braces, walk with crutches, propel wheelchairs, or navigate while blindfolded. Such experiences should be coupled with information concerning common misconceptions about and proper attitudes toward various forms of handicap. Reflex responses to painful stimuli are also easily reproduced. The dangers confronted by patients lacking pain sensations can be better appreciated after such experience. The senses of taste and smell can be easily triggered, and the decreased sense of taste that results from smoking can thereby be emphasized.

Both sensory and motor paralysis can be safely attained by applying a blood-pressure cuff or tourniquet to an arm or leg for ten or fifteen minutes. The loss of sensation and the loss of motor power is quite impressive. The tingling sensation of hyperexcitable nerves is pronounced when blood supply is restored. The kind of ischemic pain associated with coronary attacks can be simulated by having individuals exercise their arm or leg muscles when the blood supply is arrested. Students can easily listen to heart sounds, murmurs, and breath sounds with cheap stethoscopes. The origins and significance of sounds and murmurs from the

heart are no more complicated or mysterious than the physical and
chemical problems high-school students encompass today. The changes in
blood-vessel response in the skin are very easy to produce by simply
stroking the skin and watching the changes in color (triple response). A
good deal of interesting information about the function of the very smallest
blood vessels can be elicited by this simple procedure. Electrocardiographs
are rather expensive, but they are very common and could be displayed as
a demonstration (on loan) to acquaint students with the origins and simple
interpretation of such records.

Respiratory disturbances can be induced by breathing through a length
of tubing or by breathing through an obstruction. By such maneuvers the
symptoms of dyspnea and of asthma are simulated. Very simple and
inexpensive breathing tests can be performed with simple spirometers
producing data equivalent to tests conducted in clinical laboratories.

Preparation for Parenthood
From the viewpoint of society as a whole, the most important role an
individual undertakes in his lifetime is that of parent, for which society
provides and requires far less training than it does for the role of barber or
manicurist. Young people with no more basis than their own experience
often find themselves suddenly responsible for the management of a home
and the upbringing of children. The problems they face are compounded
by smaller families with fewer brothers and sisters, less responsibility of the
youth, weakening marriage ties, and rapidly changing mores. One
approach to alleviating this problem is a new educational program
sponsored by the Office of Child Development of HEW to help teenagers
prepare for parenthood by working directly with young children. Part of
the impetus for this program came from an appreciation of the statistic
that some 210,000 girls under 17 became mothers in 1971 (1 out of every
10 girls). The course, called Exploring Childhood, consists of both
classroom learning about child development and active participation in
child-care centers under the observation of teachers and parents. This
innovative concept, currently being field-tested by the Education
Development Center in Cambridge, Massachusetts, certainly deserves
consideration for expansion of scope and distribution.

Cumulative Personal Health Records

Health information is collected from any individual on an enormous number of occasions during a lifetime. Family history, past history, current health status, and clinical or laboratory data are elicited and recorded not only when a person presents signs or symptoms of illness, but also repetitively in well-baby clinics, school examinations, and applications for athletics, camps, jobs, insurance, etc. These medical records are maintained in doctors' offices, hospitals, and other institutions. With modern mobility this means that an individual's records are so dispersed as to be relatively useless. If the essential information could be selectively recorded in standard ways[9] and maintained as a cumulative personal health record, it would not only save untold waste of time and effort, but would also provide a valuable data base in case of significant illness.

In the United States this concept would be most acceptable if the records were kept only in the individual's possession. A less palatable feasibility study, from the American viewpoint, collects data from the 1.5 million people of Stockholm County into a single, mammoth computer.[10] The basic computer file on each person consists of vital statistics such as birthplace, home address, occupation, civil status, and military service, and critical medical information such as blood type, immunizations, past critical diseases, information from previous hospitalizations, previous x-ray examinations, and accumulated outpatient care. This represents an enormous feasibility study regarding the potential benefits, limitations, and unexpected complications of having such information from a total regional population available for immediate recall from many different terminals in the county.

The instant availability of this assortment of information represents an enormous investment of resources, and its overall benefits have yet to be evaluated. The possible invasion of privacy it implies is much more readily accepted in a country like Sweden where the people are more accustomed to regimentation than are citizens of the United States. There is little prospect that Americans would submit easily to having detailed information about their personal and medical past so readily accessible.

However, less reaction might be encountered if this type of information were collected and maintained in the individual's possession.

One alternative is to develop a health-data record that can be initiated by each individual during his secondary education and then maintained by him throughout his lifetime. This may seem impractical at first, but people in all walks of life are expected to be able to produce on demand their driver's license, social-security number, income-tax information, and automobile registration and title. Why not health records?

Computers and other information-handling techniques have demonstrated value in the acquisition, storage, and retrieval of medical data. Of greatest importance is the insight computer studies can give into the types and format of information that yield greatest value. For example, 75 systems for the acquisition of the history data base have been evaluated by Stephen Yarnall and Jay Wakefield.[11] Included among these techniques are a selection that are self-administered by the patient using standard forms, card-sorting, or more sophisticated computer techniques. From such efforts greatly increased insight is being gained about what information is essential, what is important, and what is desirable. Given such priorities, it becomes increasingly possible to select the content of a cumulative data base that would be applicable to much or all of the population.

The information maintained in an individual data base need not be nearly so inclusive as that which is normally maintained in a hospital record. However, sufficient selectivity should be exercised so that this self-maintained record conveys the kind of information that is regularly sought during a routine encounter with health professionals. This information could then be kept up-to-date and presented on those occasions that now call for repeated medical histories and physical examinations.

Cumulative Family and Personal Health Profiles
The traditional first stage of any history and physical examination is the recording of "pertinent data" regarding the individual's family and personal health history. This information is called for with varying degrees of completeness on innumerable occasions. Taxing the memory would not be necessary on such occasions if these data were entered on a standard

form and retained within the possession of each individual. The initiation of such forms could, for example, be made a central part of the sequence of health courses in high school. This part of the course could be coupled with instruction on the nature, source, and significance of signs and symptoms as suggested in previous sections. A carefully structured class exercise in the proper recording of the family and personal history could easily be imagined as producing a carefully completed document like that illustrated in Figure 8.4.

The first form could cover the family and past history of each individual as of age 16 or 17, with provision for additional information to be added as the occasion warrants. An incentive for individuals to keep these records up-to-date and available could be provided by means of favorable health insurance rates, not unlike the preferential treatment available to careful drivers in their accident insurance. Alternatively a rather stiff charge for re-collecting of the information by health professionals might also be effective. In addition to the personal profile and family history a set of three additional forms could be developed for the cumulative acquisition and storage of such information as: (1) the sequence of significant illnesses; (2) a list of health problems; (3) accumulated clinical data and a laboratory data profile (see Figure 8.5).

Sequential Health-Problem List

The traditional format of medical records has been challenged in recent years by Lawrence Weed, who has championed a new approach commonly known as the Problem-Oriented Medical Record.[11] This approach is designed to provide a more logical and useful mechanism for collecting, organizing, and utilizing health information so that the management of a patient's illness can be more clearly portrayed to the various members of the health team. As adopted in medical practice, the Problem-Oriented Medical Record (POMR) consists of four main components: (1) a screening data base; (2) a problem list; (3) a plan of treatment; and (4) progress notes. As an illustrative example it is possible to conceive of a modification of this approach as the basis for an individual health record such as is shown in Figure 8.5. The information regarding the past health history of the family and of the patient would correspond to the screening data base. A sequential listing of all significant health

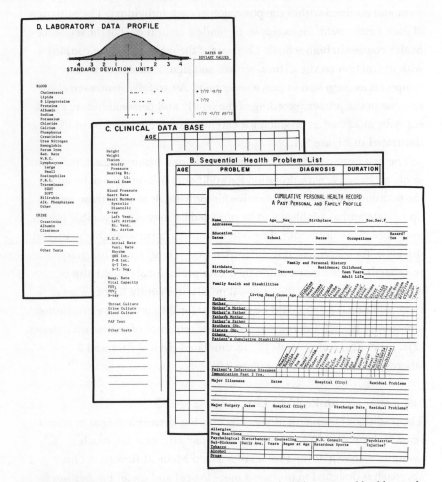

Figure 8.4 To illustrate how medical data might be accumulated in a personal health record these four forms were developed (but never actually evaluated). If cumulative health records were initiated in high school and additional entries were made during successive illnesses and testing, a comprehensive personal data base would result. The laboratory data profile is based on the concept of a standardized method of recording data (standard deviation units) to facilitate detection of deviations from the individual's normal range.[12]

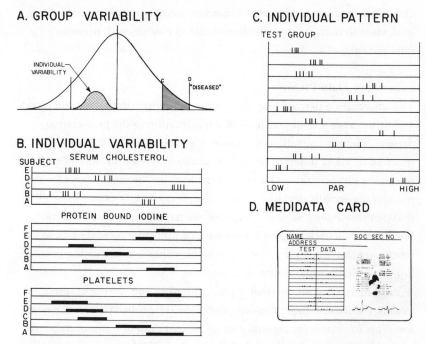

Figure 8.5 A. Laboratory test results from large groups have greater variability than data from individuals. B. Specific test results from different subjects illustrate how the individual values tend to become grouped in relatively narrow ranges. C. Test data for individual patients could be stored compactly by means of simple notations to provide distinctive patterns for reference in case of illness or disease. D. Data-packing techniques have developed to the point that a very large quantity of information can be stored on a card no larger than a driver's license and carried on the person to be readily available in case of illness or accident. From Robert F. Rushmer, *Medical Engineering* (New York: Academic Press, 1970), with permission of the publisher.

problems (signs and/or symptoms), diagnoses (if known), and durations would correspond to the problem list of the POMR. Properly filled out, this list would quickly provide a physician with the essential points of an individual's past history of health problems.

Clinical Data Base

Information collected on each subsequent contact with health professionals could be entered into a cumulative record such as that illustrated as Form C in Figure 8.5. It might be arranged so that it is necessary to insert specific or quantitative data only if there are significant deviations from preceding determinations. Simple notations could easily be devised to indicate that the data obtained concurs with previous information.

Laboratory Data Profile

The information derived from the profusion of quantitative tests on blood and urine poses serious problems of interpretation to the physician at present. The concentration of various constituents of the blood are reported in many different units. In evaluating the significance of each test result, the physician must know both the average "normal" value for the test and the specific deviations due to age, sex, and laboratory variability that determine the "normal" range for the patient under consideration. For this reason each test result calls for a complicated mental exercise in estimating the probability that a particular value is either within normal limits, outside normal limits, or borderline.

With increasing automation of clinical testing and the use of computers to store the data, sufficient information should be collected over the next few years to permit the recording of all patient data in terms of standard units.[12] Such a unit, which might be termed an SDU (standard deviation unit), would indicate the extent to which a particular value deviates from the average for the age, sex, and laboratory testing circumstances of the particular patient. If these normal values can be established and widely accepted, the process of storing enormous quantities of valuable laboratory data in readily interpreted ways will be enormously enhanced. One example is illustrated schematically as the Laboratory Data Profile (Form D, Figure 8.4).

With the advent of automation in clinical laboratories, it is almost as easy and cheap to order twelve or more tests of blood constituents as to request only one. For this reason the quantity of data collected in such routine examinations has become quite fantastic among those citizens who have access to health care. The usefulness of all of these data is limited by two major factors. First, the data is stored where taken and is therefore as widely scattered as are the histories and physical examinations. Second, the data is judged by comparison to the rather wide range of values encountered among normal individuals. Because of a combination of individual variability and differences in measurement techniques, the range of normal is very wide.

In contrast the range of normality is very much more limited for a single individual than it is for a large group. The large bell-shaped curve in Figure 8.5A represents the distribution of normal values for a group, and the small bell figure indicates the range of variability for a single individual while normal. This means that the significance and usefulness of laboratory tests can be enormously enhanced if the results can be compared with previously collected normal values *from the same individual*. This is the basic principle underlying the concept of obtaining and maintaining "profiles" of data from individuals while they are normal to serve as control baselines in case they become ill. The individual pattern of determinations is illustrated by the groups of vertical lines in Figure 8.5C, plotted from data by G.Z. Williams.[13] If each successive laboratory test result is added as collected, a "profile" would result that could be easily stored in a compact, portable form (Figure 8.5D).

Data Packing for Convenient Storage (Medidata Card)

Techniques for the miniaturization of data have been developed to a very fine art. For example, espionage agents are known to be able to reduce a page of information to a dot the size of a period (microdots). Methods are currently being used to miniaturize medical data for storage on microfiche, a degree of reduction less demanding than the microdot. In any event it is clear that a very large quantity of data could be compressed into an area no larger than a driver's license and could therefore be carried at all times. On the card schematically illustrated in Figure 8.5D sample electrocardiographic tracings are indicated at the bottom. When a patient has a sudden myocardial infarction and no previous control records are available, there is considerable uncertainty at first regarding the extent to which the wave forms have been altered from a normal control. If every citizen had a readily available reproduction of his normal ECG, such changes could be detected with very much greater clinical sensitivity. The same statement is applicable to chest x-rays, but here the process of miniaturization might pose somewhat more difficult problems. The basic concept is of particular importance, namely, cumulating information regarding significant abnormal occurrences and findings on each individual in a readily available form so reduced in size that it can be always available.

Attractive Alternatives for Lifelong Health Education

The preceding sections have presented potential opportunities for the enlightenment of young people regarding the most common and critical types of historical, physical, and laboratory information during the normal school years. Some of this indoctrination should be required during the last year(s) of legally required school attendance so that it will become widely generalized to the entire population with the passage of time. However, "one-time-through" education seems to have little lasting quality and must be reinforced with subsequent exposure at appropriate times.

Unfortunately the general public has not proved particularly receptive to educational programs presented by the mass media. If, however, the initial exposure to physiological functions, signs and symptoms of disease, and related subjects were to be rendered interesting, exciting, and relevant, the opportunities to present additional programming would be broadened. An expanding utilization of authoritative medical information in such popular television programs as the *Marcus Welby, M.D.* series is clearly one way to go. Such programs might be sponsored and supervised by recognized medical authorities. Hopefully the priorities might be set and the presentations planned to provide information useful to people who are willing and able to engage in self-care. Carefully conceived documentaries on health and health problems produced with sufficient skill to attract public interest should be utilized as much as possible. National Health Information Quiz programs in which the public is challenged to answer factual questions regarding important health issues also appear to be an appropriate format. (A familiar prototype was the National Driving Safety Quiz.) On educational television medically oriented programs with a debate format like that of *The Advocates* to consider the various aspects of significant medical problems could be promoted. For example, the issues of priorities considered in Chapter 4 lend themselves to advocacy. Ethical problems and social and economic consequences of expensive artificial organs (artificial kidneys and sophisticated artificial extremities) also represent potential subjects for multifaceted discussions.

Information of general interest is available about many different topics such as the weather, stock prices, and news from all over the world. However, if one wishes to learn the symptoms of the current "flu" epidemic, this information generally requires a call to a physician. Our massive communications network is not even being explored to determine what useful role it might play in dispensing such information to the public. Many television stations offer telecourses for university credit, but these are also frequently presented at inconvenient times. With increasing pressure for public-service programming by the FCC and with some improvement in the interest levels of such courses, they might begin to appear at more convenient times. It is fervently hoped that at least some of these could make substantial contributions to the public's understanding of health problems.

A more recent trend is the printing of college courses in newspapers. The University of California at San Diego introduced college-level courses sponsored by the National Endowment for the Humanities. The first topic was "America and the Future of Man," focusing on the impact of technology. Because of an enthusiastic response from newspapers and colleges, this prototype is now being offered more widely. The possibility of a similar course focusing on health and physiology should be vigorously explored.

Sickness: A Stimulus for Health Education

The average American exhibits little interest in gaining information about health and disease unless some kind of illness is directly affecting him or his family. If this observation is valid, opportunities should be seized to present to patients information relevant to their particular disability and general health status at those times when they are most susceptible. Physicians have always served this role, particularly when there were plenty of family doctors. Today there is a clear need for more readily available sources of information.

The time spent by patients in hospital waiting rooms, in doctors' offices, and in hospital beds might be utilized to present factual information about problems in both the patient sector and the medical sector. This might be done through videotape cassettes. Such programs might be presented with a high level of individuality once assortments of wide enough scope become available. Obviously printed matter is also still useful in this context.

Since people often go directly to a pharmacy to obtain remedies for mini-mals or common ills, there would be merit in requiring pharmaceutical companies to enclose with their products information about such subjects as side effects and drug interactions with other common drugs. It would be helpful if pharmacists were to insist that their clients know the information is there and to encourage reading it. Enclosures could include information about the illness being treated, the possible complications, the signs of such complications, and the point at which medical advice should be sought. Going one step further, medically approved kits could be generated, containing complete and authoritative information required to treat certain limited illnesses along with expert advice regarding signs, symptoms, prognosis limitations, and evidence calling for guidance by health professionals.

Summary

A successful expansion of health education could serve to reduce the tedious and unrewarding routines that plague the health system and free members of the health-care team to perform the important and sophisticated functions for which they have been so extensively trained. Patients are currently effective in the management of many health problems requiring both judgment and skill. For example, diabetics are taught to inject their own insulin and to regulate their dosages and diets to maintain themselves in balance. This is largely an individual effort under the direction of physicians.

Those illnesses that occur with highest frequency are to be found in the patient sector (mini-mals, common ills, and sui-sickness), and most of these derive little benefit from the ministrations of health professionals. Medical management of head colds or "flu" and similar mild disturbances is not very rewarding to the health professionals and not very useful to the patient. As massively expanded third-party payments in the form of national health insurance make medical care apparently free or artificially cheap, the danger of flooding the health-care system is very real. Under these conditions those patients who have serious need for access to health personnel and facilities might well find necessary care delayed or denied. Well-informed patients can improve the utilization of health-care resources. Every reasonable effort should therefore be made to encourage an improved self-care capability for as large a segment of the population as possible.

Our massive communications network has an important role to play in discouraging sui-sickness through organized efforts to combat the use of tobacco, alcohol, and drugs and to reduce the impact of such self-inflicted hazards as overeating, careless driving, and participation in hazardous sports. In this effort society must share responsibility with the individual. The management of mini-mals and common ills can be best accomplished by self-care, particularly if the general public can be supplied with the most effective drugs and with reliable information about them through proper action of the Food and Drug Administration.

Intensive indoctrination of expectant parents should be aimed at improving the effectiveness of their subsequent observation of their children for the kinds of developmental or acquired illnesses that require prompt medical attention.

Finally, if reliable and useful information is presented to individuals as an ongoing process throughout their lifetimes, a large part of the public could become effective partners in health care. One potential goal would be to expand the proportion of the public who could serve as *physicians' aides* in the management of their own illnesses, including those falling into the medical or societal categories.

References

1. *Social Forces and the Nation's Health.* 1968. Washington, D. C.: Health Services and Mental Health Administration, USPHS, HEW.
2. Nicholas Johnson. 1972. *Test Pattern for Living.* New York: Bantam Books.
3. Anne Somers. 1971. *Health Care in Transition: Directions for the Future.* Chicago: Hospital Research and Educational Trust.
4. Paul B. Cornely. 1972. National planning for health: Structure and goals. *Bull. N. Y. Acad. Med.* 48: 53–57.
5. Lewis Thomas. 1972. Your very good health. *New Eng. J. Med.* 287: 761–762.
6. S.T. Bain and W.B. Spaulding. 1967. The importance of coding presenting symptoms. *Can. Med. Assoc. J.* 97: 953–959.

7. Steven J. Englander and Charles R. Strotz. 1970. *Correlation Between Risk Factors and Subsequent Infant Morbidity.* Tucson, Ariz.: Indian Health Service, Office of Management Information Systems, Health Programs Systems Center.

8. *Children and Youth: Selected Health Characteristics U. S. 1958–1968.* National Center for Health Statistics, series 10, no. 62. Washington, D. C.: Health Services and Mental Health Administration, USPHS, HEW.

9. Lawrence L. Weed. 1968. Medical records that guide and teach. *New Eng. J. Med.* 278: 593–600, 652–657.

10. S. Abrahamsson, S. Bergstrom, K. Larsson, and S. Tillman. 1970. Danderyd Hospital computer. II. Total regional system for medical care. *Comput. Biomed. Res.* 3: 30–46.

11. Stephen R. Yarnall and Jay S. Wakefield. *Acquisition of the History Database.* 2nd ed. Seattle: Medical Computer Services Association.

12. Robert F. Rushmer. 1968. Accentuate the positive: A display system for clinical laboratory data. *J. Am. Med. Assoc.* 206: 836–838.

13. G.Z. Williams. 1962. Clinical pathology tomorrow. *Am. J. Clin. Path.* 37: 121–124.

Index